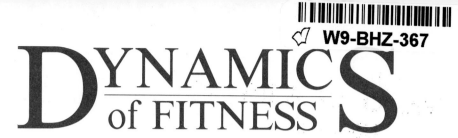

DYNAMICS
of FITNESS
A Practical Approach

George McGlynn
University of San Francisco

wcb

Wm. C. Brown Publishers
Dubuque, Iowa

Book Team

Ed Jaffe, Executive Editor
Brenda Flemming Roesch, Editor
Raphael Kadushin, Assistant Editor
Michael Warrell, Designer
Reneé Pins, Art Production Assistant
Vickie Putman Caughron, Production Editor
Faye M. Schilling, Photo Research Editor
Vicki Krug, Permissions Editor

wcb group

Wm. C. Brown, Chairman of the Board
Mark C. Falb, President and Chief Executive Officer

wcb

Wm. C. Brown Publishers, College Division

G. Franklin Lewis, Executive Vice-President, General Manager
E. F. Jogerst, Vice-President, Cost Analyst
Chris C. Guzzardo, Vice-President, Director of Marketing
George Wm. Bergquist, Editor in Chief
Beverly Kolz, Director of Production
Bob McLaughlin, National Sales Manager
Craig S. Marty, Director of Marketing Research
Marilyn A. Phelps, Manager of Design
Eugenia M. Collins, Production Editorial Manager
Faye M. Schilling, Photo Research Manager

Cover photograph © Ken Sabatini, Los Angeles, CA

To my wife, Ingeborg, and my son, George

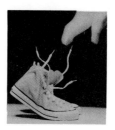

Contents

Chapter 5
Cardiovascular Fitness 63

Chapter 6
Starting Your Cardiovascular Fitness Program 77

Chapter 8
Competitive Sports and Advanced Fitness 121

Chapter 9
Nutrition and Weight Control 131

Chapter 10
Special Considerations 159

Chapter 11
Coronary Heart Disease and Exercise 179

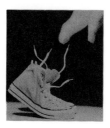

Preface

In the last few years, there have been major and widespread changes in the exercise and fitness habits of the American people. Physical health and nutrition appear to have gained a place of high priority in the scheme of everyday living. Millions of individuals are now actively engaged in marathon running, jogging, tennis, weight programs, and a variety of other rigorous physical activities. Exercise centers, sports clubs, running groups, and corporate fitness programs have proliferated and become an integral part of our social life.

Keeping pace with these changes are major scientific advances in exercise physiology and sports medicine. A great deal of knowledge presently is available in such diverse areas as training and conditioning techniques, heart disease and exercise, and muscle physiology and nutrition, to mention only a few. Unfortunately, it is very difficult for the average layperson to sift through thousands of research papers and academic volumes on sports physiology to find reliable answers to questions concerning fitness, exercise, and nutrition. My own experience as a researcher and professor of exercise physiology for over twenty-five years has supported my belief that it is important to provide information in a manner that is relevant, reliable, and understandable to rebut the misconceptions and confusion surrounding fitness and exercise. Ignorance about problems concerning exercise may not only result in wasted effort or temporary injury; in some cases, it also may lead to serious long-term health consequences. I have been constantly appalled at the health-spa, diet-book mentality that appears to dominate the popular media and continues to elevate the level of ignorance in this important area.

The purpose of this text is to provide a simple, logical, and individualized approach to developing and maintaining a high level of physical fitness. The text is intended as a practical and simple guide for understanding and evaluating your exercise needs and developing a fitness program. The information presented here represents a consensus of presently available scientific evidence in the area of exercise physiology. This text is intended primarily for college physical fitness classes, such as aerobic conditioning, interval and circuit training, and fitness and weight reduction classes, but it also can be used for health and fitness club exercise programs.

A major concern of this text is making you aware of your present level of fitness and how that can affect you the rest of your life. A sequence of simple tests enables you to analyze your present level of fitness and to compare it to established norms for your age and sex. After helping you to evaluate your present fitness, the text provides varying intensity levels of exercise that can be adapted to your individual needs for short- or long-range fitness goals dealing with cardiovascular-efficiency, muscle strength and endurance, body composition, and flexibility. The text provides record sheets and profiles for tracking your fitness level changes. It is hoped that the material in the text will increase your level of motivation so that you become actively involved in the learning process.

The final chapters of the book deal with a variety of important factors associated with fitness, including competitive sports and advanced fitness, nutrition and weight control, common injuries, environmental exercise problems, drugs used to improve athletic performance, maintaining fitness with age, females and exercise, heart disease, and stress reduction.

Introduction

Why This Book?

This book presents exercise as an integral part of your life. If you are already involved in a regular exercise program and know your way around the track and weight room, it will add to your interest by giving you new ideas and challenges. On the other hand, if you are sedentary, out of shape, self-conscious in your swimsuit, or turning into a piece of furniture in front of your television set, then this book is also for you. So, get ready for some exciting changes in your life.

It Doesn't Have to Hurt to Get in Shape

Unfortunately, many people associate physical exercise with pain, failure, and embarrassment. They view exercise as a Spartanic ritual in which they must punish themselves physically to derive any benefit. Such a concept is probably a carryover from outdated high school athletic programs—in which the coach literally ran everybody into the ground in the name of "getting in shape"—or from those grueling early morning boot camp calisthenics that all recruits endured. Also, the popular media reinforces this erroneous concept.

Certainly, when you leave the sedentary world and enter the realm of rigorous exercise, you will experience some discomforts—mild aches and pains, a slight breathing difficulty, and a feeling of fatigue. You also undoubtedly will be confronted with the morning-after symptoms of muscle soreness and fatigue. But these discomforts are usually minor and temporary and should not be of major concern. As you continue to exercise, these symptoms of beginning an exercise program will gradually disappear. Exercise should be enjoyable and relaxing, and its by-products should not be nausea and pain. In fact, if it does "hurt" when you exercise, this is a sign of overexercise and the need to moderate your activity.

Benefits of Regular Exercise

When those who regularly exercise are asked, "How have you benefited from exercise?" the answer inevitably is, "It makes me feel a lot better."

Feeling better reflects itself in a number of ways. First of all, exercise builds and maintains physical fitness. The basis for improved fitness is an increase in the work capacity of the heart and lungs, which enables the body to meet effectively those emergency conditions that require intense physical effort. This increased work capacity also provides a good physical foundation for the development of skills in a variety of sports.

It recently has been proposed that exercise may act to balance or stabilize the physiological consequences of emotional stress. Although the physiological mechanism is not yet known for certain, there is evidence of changes in hormones, neurotransmitters, and other body chemistry that may possibly help to prepare the body's response to stress situations.

For instance, increases in blood amines, glucose, androgens, lactic acid, and corticoid compounds resulting from exercise have been noted in recent research. Other evidence suggests that exercise causes the release of such chemicals as enkephalin, a euphoria-producing substance, and that physical conditioning programs facilitate the release from brain cells of beta-endorphin, a substance that produces relaxation. Some researchers attribute the beneficial effects of exercise on stress to reduced electrical activity in the muscles and an increased feeling of fitness. In combination, these factors may help to improve your self-concept, reduce your anxiety, insulate you from stress, and enhance your psychological functioning. (See chapter 12 for special stress-reduction exercises.)

Additional benefits of physical exercise are a possible delay in the aging process, protection from lower-back problems, the maintenance of body weight, and a possible reduction of the risk of coronary heart disease. Exercise also induces natural fatigue and relaxation and in some cases reduces a person's reliance on drugs that promote sleep. Finally, if you maintain good physical fitness levels, you will experience both the joy of participation in an intrinsically pleasing activity and the sense of well-being familiar to all who are involved in rigorous exercise. The most important benefit is that you not only feel good about your body, but about yourself as a human being.

To summarize, the benefits of regular exercise include:

1. Improved psychological functioning
2. Improved appearance
3. Increased efficiency of the heart and lungs
4. Increased muscle strength and endurance
5. Reduced stress response
6. Protection from lower-back problems
7. Possible delay in the aging process

8. Maintenance of proper body weight
9. Possible reduction of the risk of coronary heart disease
10. Naturally induced fatigue and relaxation

Recent Changes in the Fitness Environment

A revolution has occurred on the exercise scene during the last ten years. Today, hundreds of thousands of individuals are engaged in fitness activities. An incredible transformation in sports participation has taken place! Almost half of all adults are now engaged in some type of fitness program. Close to forty million people are jogging today. Twelve years ago, there were ten marathons in the United States and a few hundred dedicated runners. Today, there are about two hundred marathons and thousands of competitive runners. Activities such as hiking, orienteering, rafting, climbing, cross-country skiing, and scuba diving have attracted thousands.

The social and physical environments today are much different than they were twenty years ago. The mass media—in particular, television—have had a major impact on our fitness habits by giving more coverage not only to the more popular spectator sports, but also to such sports as marathon running, skiing, swimming, and cycling. In addition, there has been an astronomical rise in the general public's participation in tennis, racquetball, corporate fitness programs, aerobic dance programs, and health, running, and bicycling clubs. All of these factors have heightened most people's interest in health, nutrition, and physical fitness.

Women's participation in rigorous physical activities also has undergone marked changes in the last ten years. Traditionally, competitive sports and other physical activities were organized around male needs. Often, women were not welcome, and those who chose to participate were stigmatized by society. Because of society's rejection of this outmoded stereotype, changes in the perception of the female role, and federal legislation, hundreds of thousands of young girls and women now are actively engaged in a wide variety of rigorous physical activities. In addition, the National Organization for Women and other support groups have given strong political and emotional support to women, encouraging them to feel good—not anxious—about being physically active and competitive.

The traditional view of exercise as physically exhausting and boring has been replaced by the contemporary view of it as enjoyable, healthful, and beneficial. Today, free of the demands of high-level skills or the fear of failure and ridicule, almost anyone can identify himself or herself as an athlete by just putting on running shoes and shorts and heading for the jogging trail.

Participation has taken priority over spectating. You definitely gain a much more authentic experience from participating in physical activities than from watching others. More and more people are themselves experiencing for the first time the joy, the satisfaction, the sense of accomplishment, and yes, even the pain and sometimes the failure of those who participate.

A more abstract, but nevertheless valuable, view of participation deals with the unique nature of the values accorded to this experience by those who participate. Existentialist philosopher Albert Camus once said that it is only the individual who gives value to life, that knowledge is a personal thing, and that the world is silent and irrational and yields no answer to us in our quest to know. According to Camus, whatever you experience depends upon your own individual perception. Thus, you are as old as you feel; the taste of vanilla ice cream is unique to each person; running, swimming, and hiking are experienced differently by each individual; and a song, a poem, a victory, or a defeat means whatever you think it does.

Our misconceptions about fitness are legends that persist despite recent change. Many people still find it surprising that professional athletes, such as baseball players and golfers, may have poor cardiovascular fitness. Some still expect that fitness automatically will be conferred upon them just because their work requires some physical exertion, such as lifting or moving. Others feel that bouncing, vibrating, and whirlpooling their muscles in a health spa are the shortest ways to fitness. These obvious misconceptions may stem partly from two varying definitions of fitness: performance-related fitness and health-related fitness.

Performance-Related Versus Health-Related Fitness

Performance-related fitness relates to many of the tests you may have taken, usually in schools, that measured your levels of strength, skill, power, endurance, and agility in specific sports. These are performance-related tests and measure only limited aspects of fitness.

The main goal of this book is to develop the concept of **health-related fitness,** which concerns those aspects of our physical and psychological makeup that afford us some protection against coronary heart disease, problems associated with being overweight, a variety of muscle and joint ailments, and the physiological complications of our responses to stress.

The President's Council on Physical Fitness and Sports more comprehensively defines health-related fitness as the ability to carry out daily tasks with vigor, without undue fatigue, and with ample energy to enjoy leisure-time pursuits and to meet unforeseen injuries. This definition indicates that fitness is a relative term relating to your everyday activities. For example, some of us may have occupations that require higher levels of fitness than others (a construction worker compared to a secretary for instance), but all individuals must meet a minimum level of fitness to lead a healthy and productive life.

The four components of health-related fitness that are essential to leading a healthy life are cardiovascular efficiency, muscle strength and endurance, body composition, and flexibility.

Cardiovascular Efficiency

At the heart of physical fitness is **cardiovascular efficiency,** which is the body's ability to deliver oxygen to all of its vital organs. How well the body provides oxygen is determined primarily by the efficiency of the heart and respiratory system. The cardiovascular system must be able to transport oxygen efficiently to provide energy to the heart, nervous system, and working muscles. When insufficient oxygen is delivered to the muscles, their capacity to do work sharply declines. A heart in excellent condition and an efficient respiratory system are essential to a high level of physical fitness. Exercise increases the strength of the heart, which increases its ability to pump blood more efficiently throughout the body. One of the main benefits of this is the potential for increasing the supply of oxygen to the heart muscle itself. Exercise also results in the reduction of epinephrine production, heart rate, and blood pressure. When these three factors are reduced at rest, the amount of oxygen needed by the heart muscle is reduced.

In the past few years, there have been major advances in the research on heart disease and its relationship to exercise. Studies of the physiological adjustments and the demands made upon the heart during exercise have provided a basis for stress-testing programs. As a result, individualized exercise and rehabilitation programs have been adapted to the needs of those who are predisposed to or who have coronary heart disease. Not long ago, when individuals suffered a heart attack, they were told to avoid exercise for fear of further injury to the heart. More recent research has now shown that exercise can be extremely beneficial to certain individuals who have suffered heart attacks. In fact, individually prescribed exercise programs may increase the efficiency of the heart to the point where it is possible to improve the circulation and reduce the risk of subsequent heart attacks.

The American Heart Association Committee on Exercise advocates physical activity as an adjunct to the control of blood pressure, blood lipid levels, and obesity. In recommending individualized exercise programs, the committee states that "exercise can enrich the quality of life and in combination with other measures, such as low-fat diets and eliminating smoking, can help reduce coronary risk, and that exercise is the most significant factor contributing to the health of the individual."*

Muscle Strength and Endurance

Muscle strength is the force produced when a muscle group is in the process of lifting, moving, or pushing a resistance. Strength is essential to a variety of everyday activities. Even though muscle strength is a relative factor related to the demand of the activity, a minimum level of strength is needed by all individuals. Those with lower levels of strength run a greater risk of injury when lifting

*American Heart Association Subcommittee on Exercise and Cardiac Rehabilitation, "Statement on Exercise," *Circulation* 64(1981):1302–4.

or engaging in physical activities. Performance in recreational sports and athletics is enhanced by higher levels of strength. Power, the ability of the muscle to produce high levels of force in a short period of time, is also basic to a number of daily activities.

Strong abdominal muscles are an important component of body fitness. The abdominal muscles, for example, form a strong support for your internal organs. These organs exert considerable stress against the inner surface of the abdominal muscles. The more stretched the muscles become, as in the case of a protruding abdomen, the more heavily the internal organs press against the abdominal wall. Visceroptosis is a condition in which abdominal protrusion is so severe that the viscera (internal organs) drop down into new positions. The stomach, liver, spleen, kidneys, and intestines all may be displaced, adversely affecting their functions. This forward displacement of the abdominal wall and the visceral contents is due to a lack of abdominal muscle strength. Adequate contraction of the abdominal muscles also prevents the muscles in the lower back from reversing their normal function and hyperextending the lumbar spin (that is, inward arching). Hyperextension can result in additional pressure on the spinal discs, which could cause pain and chronic injury.

As we grow older, we all incur losses in muscle strength. However, those who maintain a strength program can delay these losses. In addition, a strength program maintains greater maximum strength for dealing efficiently with everyday physical activities and sudden emergencies. Better posture accompanied by a more aesthetic appearance are also benefits of strength maintenance.

Body Composition

Body composition refers to the proportion of body fat to lean body tissue. The relative balance of these two body components is a better gauge of fitness level than ordinary body weight. A recommended proportion of body fat for a man in his early twenties is approximately 15 percent; for a woman in the same age group, about 26 percent is recommended.

Obesity is one of the most important health problems confronting Americans today. Approximately 20 percent of the teenage population, 30 percent of all men, and 40 percent of all women weigh 15 to 20 percent more than they should. Obesity has important ramifications to health. Being overweight is one of the major risk factors associated with heart disease. Diabetes and high blood pressure generally accompany being overweight, and exercise accompanied by weight loss can directly affect these two common problems. Obesity is also associated with gallbladder dysfunction, joint disease, and complications during surgery.

When you exercise, you inevitably burn up more calories than when you are sedentary; therefore, you start to lose weight, provided your food intake remains the same. An exercise program may result in an increase of muscle tissue with a decrease in stored fat. Because muscles weigh more than fat, you may actually gain a little weight even though you undergo a loss in body fat. Your body dimensions, however, will change, resulting in a slim waist, trim hips and thighs, and an improved overall appearance.

Flexibility

Flexibility is the movement of a joint through the full range of motion. Flexibility is important not only to learning athletic skills satisfactorily but also to general health and fitness. A decreased range of motion may limit proper movement and lead to inefficient movement as well as to the possibility of injury to ligaments and tendons.

How Long before Results Show Up?

Now that you know what fitness is all about, be patient. Fitness is not developed in a few days, so give yourself some time. However, after only a few weeks, you should begin to feel some physical changes, such as less breathlessness and fatigue. If you have been sedentary for a number of years, you should not expect to sense responses within a few weeks. Your body will take a number of months to adjust to the demands of exercise in order to gear up for increases in efficiency. Don't expect miracles to occur in a few weeks. Convince yourself that it will be necessary to invest a lot of time in training. Research indicates that people engaged in a rigorous physical exercise program start to experience increased efficiency in the cardiovascular system in approximately eight weeks, and progressive increases follow thereafter. There are also many individual differences that affect each person's responsiveness to training—age, sex, race, genetic disposition, exercise history, medical history, and motivation all play an important part.

Exercises to Avoid

Some exercises that have been popular in the past may be harmful and should be avoided. First of all, you should never end an exercise period with a wind sprint. Running to exhaustion at the end of exercise is unnecessary and can have a dangerous effect upon the heart. Taper off very slowly when ending exercise. Such exercises as deep-knee bends, walking with your knees bent (duck walk), and holding the knee partially flexed for periods of time can cause stress and injury to the knee joint. Toe touching, which some people use to stretch their hamstring muscles, can cause injury to the lower back. Sit-up exercises with the legs straight and double leg lifts both place a lot of stress on the lower back, especially if you have weak abdominal muscles. Leg splits can be dangerous because most individuals don't have the proper flexibility for this position and may suffer damage to the muscles and tendons in the legs and groin.

If you follow the guidelines and the individualized exercises presented in this book, you will be following procedures based upon sound scientific principles, which will not only benefit your health, but also be a source of continued enjoyment to you.

Key Terms

Body Composition   The proportion of body fat to lean body tissue

Cardiovascular Efficiency   The ability of the heart to deliver oxygen to all of the vital organs of the body

Flexibility   The extent and range of motion around a joint

Health-Related Fitness   Those aspects of our physical and psychological makeup that afford us some protection against coronary heart disease, problems associated with being overweight, muscle and joint ailments, and the physiological complications of responding to stress

Muscle Strength   The force produced by a muscle group

CHAPTER

2

Motivation

It's All Up to You

Behavior generally is motivated by a desire to attain goals that give value and meaning to our lives. **Motivation** is the energy that fuels the engines of behavior that drive toward these goals. Its presence explains why we strive, work, and persevere.

Recent research reveals that a considerable number of individuals who begin weight loss, drug rehabilitation, and similar programs drop out long before achieving much progress. Furthermore, as these programs progress, participants display decreased interest and reduce their efforts. The mainsprings of their actions appear to stop working, and they no longer are able to maintain their goal-directed activity.

Human motivation depends on a series of choices based on our perceptions. It is possible that the individuals who drop out of the previously mentioned improvement programs do value their goals but that the perceived relationships between program activity and goal achievement are uncertain, leading to reduced commitment. Generally, the force of effort maintained by individuals toward their goals is determined by two factors: their perceived chances of achieving the desired outcomes and the degree of value they place on the outcomes. In other words, each person internalizes his or her chances of success and also the value of that success to his or her well-being. ("What are my chances of losing those twenty-five pounds, and if I do lose them, of what value is that twenty-five-pound loss to me?")

Before starting an exercise program, it is important that you evaluate your present circumstances and satisfactorily answer two important questions:

1. What are my chances of increasing my overall physical fitness?
2. Will the changes brought about by exercise be of value to me?

The answer to the first question is relatively easy: Excellent. Research indicates that the low-fit or sedentary individual can look forward to substantial gains in cardiovascular and muscular fitness after only a few months of continuous, rigorous exercise.

You will have to answer the second question yourself. However, here are some thoughts to consider. If you are now sedentary, it is reasonable to assume that the physical and psychological changes discussed in chapter 1 that occur in your body as a result of exercise will be of some value to you. In addition, research indicates that we all have certain basic needs in common that must be fulfilled to lead a balanced life. For example, we all enjoy the satisfaction of achievement, whether it comes from a promotion at work or from jogging two miles without stopping. Also, knowing that we can achieve our goals is an important reinforcement of our need to experience some control over our environment. A sense of mastery, the completion of a task, or the learning of a valued skill that once seemed difficult to acquire can all lead to feelings of self-confidence and well-being. The desire to witness and control our environment, to enjoy it, to react to it, and to master it is the most significant factor in providing satisfaction. Furthermore, we gain satisfaction from meaningful activities and from opportunities to develop a sense of responsibility and self-direction. All of these needs can be met by a sound exercise program.

It's very easy to find excuses *not* to exercise. Too cold, too hot, too windy, too busy, too tired, will make it up next week—all are frequently heard. However, if you accept the goals of health-related fitness and are aware of how they relate to your self-concept, you soon will be looking for excuses *to* exercise.

Chapter 1 focused more on the physical benefits of rigorous exercise. The following are some of the more psychological and social benefits:

1. **You Don't Have to Worry about Failing.** There are no complex skills to learn, no condescending instructors, no embarrassing situations, no last-place finishes, no critical peers, no intimidation.

2. **You See Results.** You are reshaping your body. Improving your cardiovascular efficiency increases your feelings of health and energy. Moreover, weight-resistance training improves your sense of muscular strength and well-being.

3. **You Can Say Goodbye to Destructive Self-Criticism.** No racket throwing, no recriminations, no self-destructive thoughts. Certainly a progressive increase in exercise requires some adaptation of effort on your part, but what activity doesn't?

4. **You Compete Only with Yourself.** You can set your own goals and forget about peer pressure. There are no opponents to defeat, no times to overcome, no records to break.

5. **You Make All the Decisions.** You are truly master of your own fate. You can decide your own schedule and set your own rules and standards. You can exercise alone, exercise with a friend, do your own thing.

6. **You Receive Social Approval.** Everyone admires people who exercise. You may find and make new friends. You are putting yourself in a no-lose social environment.

7. **You Experience an Improved Self-Image and Recognition.** Extra inches off the waistline, increased feelings of well-being and energy, a more aesthetic looking body—these goals are all within your range of achievement.

8. **You Feel Satisfied.** Achieving goals that you personally have established, working toward more self-confidence, and getting a clear focus on your life all bring increased satisfaction.

9. **You Are Successful.** No one fails when they exercise, but don't expect a "quick fix" after only a few days. Be patient and the outcome will be positive.

10. **You Have a Chance to Express Yourself.** Exercise provides one of the few opportunities for emotional release and free expression. You be the judge of what you want to do with your body. Tune in to its signals, and you'll be surprised at what you hear.

Guidelines to Keep You Exercising

Find a Convenient Location to Work Out. Choose a place to exercise that is close to where you work or live. Don't depend on others for transportation.

Vary Your Exercises. To avoid boredom, don't get locked into one routine, whether it's warm-up, jogging, swimming, or weights. Be creative.

Stay within Your Limits. Don't set goals that leave you exhausted.

Record Your Progress. If you keep track of what's happening to your body, heart rate, strength, and weight, you will be amazed at the changes. Such records also provide great feedback and reinforcement. Appendix B at the back of the book provides record sheets for most of the exercise regimens presented in this text.

Don't Be Obsessive about Exercise. Keep records, but don't keep score. You don't have to keep piling it on. Two miles a day is a lot safer and healthier than twenty miles, and besides, it's more enjoyable.

Be Patient, and Stay with It. The benefits do not come overnight. Generally, it takes a few months for physiological changes to become noticeable.

Set Your Own Time Schedule. It is important to organize a convenient schedule. Don't make it too rigid. Allow for some flexibility.

Exercise Dependence

Now that you are ready to become exercise enthusiasts, you should be cautioned about **exercise dependence.** Would you believe that research indicates that some individuals may become addicted to or dependent on exercise? That running four or five days a week for forty-five minutes accelerates the production of **enkephalin,** a euphoria-producing substance? And that the level of intensity of the exercise must be increased to maintain that euphoric feeling? You may have seen exercise addicts in your office or on your block. They spend more time in their running shorts than in their designer jeans. They become so obsessed with setting higher and higher goals that they lose sight of the many physiological, psychological, and social benefits that exercise affords. Unfortunately, the body cannot tolerate these continued high levels of stressful exercise, and it eventually begins to break down in the form of chronic muscle soreness and inflamed tendons and joints. When an individual is forced to stop exercising because of such injuries, this deprivation from exercise may lead to symptoms similar to those of drug withdrawal. This forced abstinence from exercise also may lead to a reinforcement of a neurotic need to exercise.

This theory of exercise addiction is still debatable, but it is important nevertheless to be aware of this possibility and to view your exercise program in the context of the total fitness goals expressed in chapter 1. Don't keep score or continually strive for that euphoric feeling. Be aware of why you are out there jogging or swimming, and set reasonable goals. Don't feel guilty because you have to miss a few days of exercise. Keep your own goals in mind as you listen to peers chatter about their experiences of "runner's high" during super long distances or if peers ask condescending questions about your motivation and fitness if you are not training for the local marathon. Don't let others dictate your exercise program. If others want to set unreal, unnecessary standards for themselves—and possibly create emotional problems in the process—that's their problem. Don't let them make it yours.

The ultimate purpose of most individuals is to be themselves and to achieve the realization of their personal self-concept. We all tend to be in perpetual pursuit of what we regard as our deserved role in life and want to be treated and rewarded in relationship to our ability. When our experience confirms this, we tend to stay committed and persevere toward our goals.

Key Terms

Enkephalin   A euphoria-producing substance

Exercise Dependence   The phenomenon of possible physiological or psychological addiction to exercise

Motivation   The basic reasons why we strive, work, and persevere toward our goals

Fitness Evaluation

Evaluating Your Fitness

The old saying, "You can't get lost if you don't know where you are going," is very appropriate to starting a fitness program. It is vital that an objective evaluation of your present fitness status be made so that the proper intensity, duration, and frequency of exercise can be prescribed. This evaluation enables you to set reasonable fitness goals and prevents unnecessary stress on your body systems.

The tests in this chapter evaluate the four basic components of physical fitness: (1) cardiovascular efficiency, (2) body composition, (3) flexibility, and (4) muscle strength and endurance. Norms are provided for each fitness component so that you are able to compare your fitness levels with the prescribed norms for your age and sex.

These tests, which have been used for a number of years, have provided thousands of individuals their first chance to assess their fitness. Because of the many variables found in fitness tests, such as sex, age, height, weight, and flexibility, these tests are not precise measures and are subject to error. With this in mind, don't overemphasize the importance of the test standards. They are to be used as general guides for the outline of your fitness program and as indicators of how you compare with other individuals of your age and sex.

Your physical fitness profile charts (tables 3.18–3.30 and figures 3.16 and 3.17) are found at the end of the chapter. When they are properly filled out, the interpretation of your profile will point out areas in need of improvement and provide the starting levels for your exercise program. You should reevaluate all of the fitness components six to eight weeks after commencing your exercise program.

Tests for Cardiovascular Fitness

The chief means of evaluating **cardiovascular efficiency** is to determine the body's capacity to consume oxygen at a maximum rate. In other words, determine the greatest amount of oxygen that can be utilized by the cells per unit of time during maximum exercise, which is referred to as the maximum oxygen uptake. The assessment of oxygen uptake through laboratory testing is accurate, but it requires a certain amount of time and sophisticated equipment, which would be impractical for determining your own fitness. Instead, there are a number of cardiovascular tests that indirectly measure the amount of maximum oxygen uptake by determining the heart rate response to certain prescribed exercises.

Five different tests are provided for you to measure your cardiovascular fitness: the 1.5-mile run, the step test, the two-minute jogging-in-place test, the bicycle ergometer test, and the swimming test. These tests, which measure the heart's response to various intensities of exercise, are good measures of your cardiovascular fitness level.

The 1.5-mile run should be attempted only by those individuals in good enough condition to run this distance. All others should use either the step test, the bicycle ergometer test, the jogging-in-place test, or the swimming test. If you cannot obtain a bench of proper height for the step test, use the jogging-in-place test. The bicycle ergometer test and the swimming test, unlike the others, are nonweight-bearing tests, which are more appropriate if you plan to cycle or swim for fitness. You also may wish to take all five tests; in this way, you have a more reliable measure of your fitness. However, you need take only *one* of the following five tests before starting your exercise program.

1.5-Mile Run

The 1.5-mile test can be run on an oval track or on a straightaway. You only should consider this test if you have been conditioned to run this distance or are in good physical condition. If you are over thirty-five years of age, you should not take this test unless you have had a stress electrocardiogram that was normal or have had a thorough physical examination. If you become overtired while running, shift down to a slow jog or walk. Do not unduly overstress yourself. Keep track of the amount of time it takes you to run the 1.5 miles, and then find your fitness level in tables 3.1 and 3.2. Record your score and fitness level on your fitness evaluation form (table 3.18).

Table 3.1 Estimated Maximum Oxygen Uptake (V̇O₂ max) for 1.5-Mile Run

Time (min:sec)	Estimated VO₂ max (ml/kg/min)	Time (min:sec)	Estimated VO₂ max (ml/kg/min)
7:30 and under	75	12:31–13:00	39
7:31–8:00	72	13:01–13:30	37
8:01–8:30	67	13:31–14:00	36
8:31–9:00	62	14:01–14:30	34
9:01–9:30	58	14:31–15:00	33
9:31–10:00	55	15:01–15:30	31
10:01–10:30	52	15:31–16:00	30
10:31–11:00	49	16:01–16:30	28
11:01–11:30	46	16:31–17:00	27
11:31–12:00	44	17:01–17:30	26
12:01–12:30	41	17:31–18:00	25

Source: From Cooper, K. H., "A means of assessing maximal oxygen uptake," in *Journal of the American Medical Association*, pp. 201–204. © 1968 American Medical Association. Reprinted by permission of the publisher.

Table 3.2 Range of Maximum Oxygen Uptake Values (ml/kg/min) with Age

Age group (years)	Fitness level						
	Very poor	Poor	Average	Good	Very good	Excellent	Superior
10–19	Below 25	25–35	35–38	38–46	47–56	57–66	Above 66
20–29	Below 24	24–31	31–33	33–42	43–52	53–62	Above 62
30–39	Below 23	23–25	25–30	30–38	39–48	49–58	Above 58
40–49	Below 21	21–23	23–26	26–35	36–44	45–54	Above 54
50–59	Below 19	19–21	21–24	24–33	34–41	42–50	Above 50
60–69	Below 18	18–20	20–22	22–30	31–38	39–46	Above 46
70–79	Below 17	17–19	19–20	20–27	28–35	36–42	Above 42

Source: From Cooper, K. H., "A means of assessing maximal oxygen uptake," in *Journal of the American Medical Association*, pp. 201–204. © 1968 American Medical Association. Reprinted by permission of the publisher.

Note: Since females are generally 20 percent lower (on average) compared to males, normal values for females can be obtained by shifting over one category to the right. For example, the "average" category for males would be considered "good" for females.

Step Test

This five-minute pulse-recovery step test consists of stepping at approximately twenty-three steps per minute for exactly five minutes.

Equipment needed for the test includes (1) a bench that is 15¾ inches (40 centimeters) high for men or 13 inches (33 centimeters) high for women and (2) a metronome or another audible signaling device (for example, a tape-recorded metronome) programmed for ninety beats per minute. Room temperature should be between sixty-eight degrees and seventy-four degrees Fahrenheit (F).

The test directions are as follows:

1. Take your resting heart rate five minutes before the test.
2. Step onto the bench with one foot (tick), then the other (tock), and return (tick, tock) in a four-count sequence. You should complete one sequence approximately every three seconds.
3. After completing five minutes of exercise, sit down and take your pulse for exactly fifteen seconds, starting exactly at fifteen seconds and ending exactly at thirty seconds after exercise. The pulse is taken by placing four fingertips in the groove directly below the base of the thumb on the underside of the wrist.
4. Weigh yourself in the clothing worn during the test.

The step test should not be given after strenuous activity, immediately after drinking coffee or smoking, or in an extremely warm room (above seventy-eight degrees Fahrenheit).

When properly administered, the step test gives an accurate estimate of your maximum oxygen intake, or physical fitness. Scores do not fluctuate even with extreme differences in resting heart rates. In addition, this test does not place undue stress on the respiratory and circulatory systems. Therefore, it is especially useful in screening individuals who are at various levels of physical fitness.

To determine your cardiovascular fitness category, refer to tables 3.3 and 3.4, which are fitness indexes for men and women, to table 3.5 for age-adjusted scores, and to table 3.6 for a fitness rating. Then record your score and fitness level on your fitness evaluation form (table 3.19).

To use the fitness indexes in tables 3.3 and 3.4, locate the number that is directly above your body weight (bottom horizontal column) and that intersects horizontally with your postexercise heart rate found in the left-hand column. Now locate this number in the top horizontal column of table 3.5. The number that is directly below this number and opposite your age is your age-adjusted score. Finally, locate your age-adjusted score opposite your age in table 3.6 to determine your fitness rating.

For example, a forty-year-old male who weighs 160 pounds and has a postexercise heart rate of 29 (per fifteen seconds) would have a score of 50 (table 3.3). A score of 50 for a forty-year-old male results in an age-adjusted score of 47 (table 3.5). The fitness rating in table 3.6 for a score of 47 is "excellent."

Table 3.3 — Fitness Index for Men

Fitness score

Postexercise pulse count	120	130	140	150	160	170	180	190	200	210	220	230	240
45	33	33	33	33	33	32	32	32	32	32	32	32	32
44	34	34	34	34	33	33	33	33	33	33	33	33	33
43	35	35	35	34	34	34	34	34	34	34	34	34	34
42	36	35	35	35	35	35	35	35	35	35	35	34	34
41	36	36	36	36	36	36	36	36	36	36	36	35	35
40	37	37	37	37	37	37	37	37	36	36	36	36	36
39	38	38	38	38	38	38	38	38	38	38	38	37	37
38	39	39	39	39	39	39	39	39	39	39	39	38	38
37	41	40	40	40	40	40	40	40	40	40	40	39	39
36	42	42	41	41	41	41	41	41	41	41	41	40	40
35	43	43	42	42	42	42	42	42	42	42	42	42	41
34	44	44	43	43	43	43	43	43	43	43	43	43	43
33	46	45	45	45	45	45	44	44	44	44	44	44	44
32	47	47	46	46	46	46	46	46	46	46	46	46	46
31	48	48	48	47	47	47	47	47	47	47	47	47	47
30	50	49	49	49	48	48	48	48	48	48	48	48	48
29	52	51	51	51	50	50	50	50	50	50	50	50	50
28	53	53	53	53	52	52	52	52	52	52	51	51	51
27	55	55	55	54	54	54	54	54	54	53	53	53	52
26	57	57	56	56	56	56	56	56	56	55	55	54	54
25	59	59	58	58	58	58	58	58	58	56	56	55	55
24	60	60	60	60	60	60	60	59	59	58	58	57	
23	62	62	61	61	61	61	61	60	60	60	59		
22	64	64	63	63	63	63	62	62	61	61			
21	66	66	65	65	65	64	64	64	62				
20	68	68	67	67	67	66	66	65					

Body weight

Source: "Step Test," by Brian Sharkey, copyright 1984, Human Kinetics Publ., Champaign, IL 61820.

| Table 3.4 | | | | Fitness Index for Women | | | | | | | |

Fitness score

Postexercise pulse count	80	90	100	110	120	130	140	150	160	170	180	190
45										29	29	29
44								30	30	30	30	30
43							31	31	31	31	31	31
42			32	32	32	32	32	32	32	32	32	32
41			33	33	33	33	33	33	33	33	33	33
40			34	34	34	34	34	34	34	34	34	34
39			35	35	35	35	35	35	35	35	35	35
38			36	36	36	36	36	36	36	36	36	36
37			37	37	37	37	37	37	37	37	37	37
36		37	38	38	38	38	38	38	38	38	38	38
35	38	38	39	39	39	39	39	39	39	39	39	39
34	39	39	40	40	40	40	40	40	40	40	40	40
33	40	40	41	41	41	41	41	41	41	41	41	41
32	41	41	42	42	42	42	42	42	42	42	42	42
31	42	42	43	43	43	43	43	43	43	43	43	43
30	43	43	44	44	44	44	44	44	44	44	44	44
29	44	44	45	45	45	45	45	45	45	45	45	45
28	45	45	46	46	46	47	47	47	47	47	47	
27	46	46	47	48	48	49	49	49	49	49		
26	47	48	49	50	50	51	51	51	51			
25	49	50	51	52	52	53	53					
24	51	52	53	54	54	55						
23	53	54	55	56	56	57						

Body weight

Source: "Step Test," by Brian Sharkey, copyright 1984, Human Kinetics Publ., Champaign, IL 61820.

Table 3.5 **Age-Adjusted Fitness Scores**

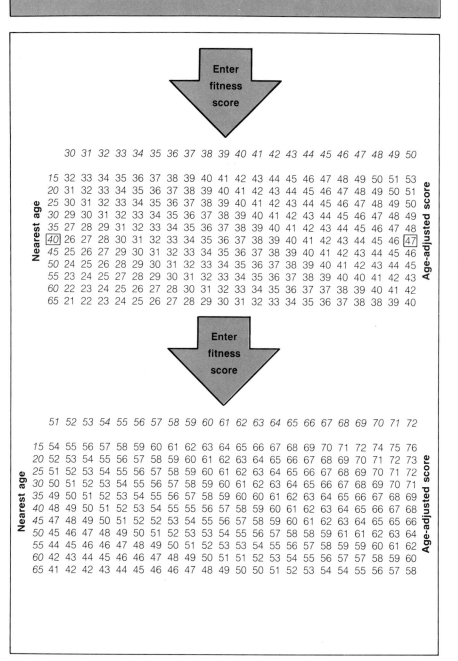

	Enter fitness score

Nearest age	30	31	32	33	34	35	36	37	38	39	40	41	42	43	44	45	46	47	48	49	50	
15	32	33	34	35	36	37	38	39	40	41	42	43	44	45	46	47	48	49	50	51	53	
20	31	32	33	34	35	36	37	38	39	40	41	42	43	44	45	46	47	48	49	50	51	
25	30	31	32	33	34	35	36	37	38	39	40	41	42	43	44	45	46	47	48	49	50	
30	29	30	31	32	33	34	35	36	37	38	39	40	41	42	43	44	45	46	47	48	49	
35	27	28	29	31	32	33	34	35	36	37	38	39	40	41	42	43	44	45	46	47	48	
40	26	27	28	30	31	32	33	34	35	36	37	38	39	40	41	42	43	44	45	46	47	
45	25	26	27	29	30	31	32	33	34	35	36	37	38	39	40	41	42	43	44	45	46	
50	24	25	26	28	29	30	31	32	33	34	35	36	37	38	39	40	41	42	43	44	45	
55	23	24	25	27	28	29	30	31	32	33	34	35	36	37	38	39	40	40	41	42	43	
60	22	23	24	25	26	27	28	30	31	32	33	34	35	36	37	37	38	39	40	41	42	
65	21	22	23	24	25	26	27	28	29	30	31	32	33	34	35	36	37	38	38	39	40	

Age-adjusted score

	Enter fitness score

Nearest age	51	52	53	54	55	56	57	58	59	60	61	62	63	64	65	66	67	68	69	70	71	72	
15	54	55	56	57	58	59	60	61	62	63	64	65	66	67	68	69	70	71	72	74	75	76	
20	52	53	54	55	56	57	58	59	60	61	62	63	64	65	66	67	68	69	70	71	72	73	
25	51	52	53	54	55	56	57	58	59	60	61	62	63	64	65	66	67	68	69	70	71	72	
30	50	51	52	53	54	55	56	57	58	59	60	61	62	63	64	65	66	67	68	69	70	71	
35	49	50	51	52	53	54	55	56	57	58	59	60	60	61	62	63	64	65	66	67	68	69	
40	48	49	50	51	52	53	54	55	55	56	57	58	59	60	61	62	63	64	65	66	67	68	
45	47	48	49	50	51	52	52	53	54	55	56	57	58	59	60	61	62	63	64	65	65	66	
50	45	46	47	48	49	50	51	52	53	53	54	55	56	57	58	58	59	61	61	62	63	64	
55	44	45	46	46	47	48	49	50	51	52	53	53	54	55	56	57	58	59	59	60	61	62	
60	42	43	44	45	46	46	47	48	49	50	51	51	52	53	54	55	56	57	57	58	59	60	
65	41	42	42	43	44	45	46	46	47	48	49	50	50	51	52	53	54	54	55	56	57	58	

Age-adjusted score

Source: "Step Test," by Brian Sharkey, copyright 1984, Human Kinetics Publ., Champaign, IL 61820.

<table>

Table 3.6	Fitness Rating of Men and Women

Physical fitness rating—men

(Use age-adjusted score)

Nearest age

Nearest age	Superior	Excellent	Very good	Good	Average	Poor	Very poor
15	57+	56-52	51-47	46-42	41-37	36-32	31-
20	56+	55-51	50-46	45-41	40-36	35-31	30-
25	55+	54-50	49-45	44-40	39-35	34-30	29-
30	54+	53-49	48-44	43-39	38-34	33-29	28-
35	53+	52-48	47-43	42-38	37-33	32-28	27-
40	52+	51-47	46-42	41-37	36-32	31-27	26-
45	51+	50-46	45-41	40-36	35-31	30-26	25-
50	50+	49-45	44-40	39-35	34-30	29-25	24-
55	49+	48-44	43-39	38-34	33-29	28-24	23-
60	48+	47-43	42-38	37-33	32-28	27-23	22-
65	47+	48-42	41-37	36-32	31-27	26-22	21-

Fitness level

Physical fitness rating—women

(Use age-adjusted score)

Nearest age

Nearest age	Superior	Excellent	Very good	Good	Average	Poor	Very poor
15	54+	53-49	48-44	43-39	38-34	33-29	28-
20	53+	52-48	47-43	42-38	37-33	32-28	27-
25	52+	51-47	46-42	41-37	36-32	31-27	26-
30	51+	50-46	45-41	40-36	35-31	30-26	25-
35	50+	49-45	44-40	39-35	34-30	29-25	24-
40	49+	48-44	43-39	38-34	33-29	28-24	23-
45	48+	47-43	42-38	37-33	32-28	27-23	22-
50	47+	46-42	41-37	36-32	31-27	26-22	21-
55	46+	45-41	40-36	35-31	30-26	25-21	20-
60	45+	44-40	39-35	34-30	29-25	24-20	19-
65	44+	43-39	38-34	33-29	28-24	23-20	19-

Fitness level

</table>

Source: "Step Test," by Brian Sharkey, copyright 1984, Human Kinetics Publ., Champaign, IL 61820.

Table 3.7 Two-Minute Jogging-in-Place Scores

Fitness level	Difference between preexercise and postexercise thirty-second pulse rate
Very poor	+15
Poor	11–14
Average	8–10
Good	6–7
Very good	4–5
Excellent	1–3
Superior	0

Two-Minute Jogging-in-Place Test

The two-minute jogging-in-place test is useful if you are unable to find a track or a measured distance to run, if your present physical condition prevents you from running 1.5 miles, or if you are unable to find an appropriate size bench for the step test.

The test directions are as follows:

1. Sit quietly for two minutes.
2. Count your pulse rate for thirty seconds and record it.
3. Jog in place for two minutes at approximately three steps per second (180 beats per minute on a metronome, at one step per beat).
4. Sit immediately after completing the two-minute jogging period, and within five seconds, take your pulse for thirty seconds.
5. Find the difference between your preexercise thirty-second pulse rate and your postexercise thirty-second pulse rate. Now find this number in table 3.7.

Record your score and fitness level on your fitness evaluation form (table 3.20).

Bicycle Ergometer Test

For those of you who have access to a bicycle ergometer (stationary bicycle), this is a simple five-minute test for measuring your aerobic fitness. The test directions are as follows:

1. The bicycle ergometer pedal speed should be set at 60 RPM (revolutions per minute) with a work load of 150 watts (900-kilopound meters per minute) for males and 100 watts (600-kilopound meters per minute) for females. Poorly conditioned individuals or those over forty years of age should exercise at a work load of 50 watts (300-kilopound meters per minute).
2. The exercise duration is five minutes. Warm up one minute with no load on the pedal before commencing the five-minute exercise.
3. Measure your heart rate for fifteen seconds during the latter half of the fifth minute.

Once you have determined your fifteen-second heart rate during the fifth minute of the exercise, find your fitness index score opposite your heart rate and underneath the appropriate work load column in table 3.8. Then locate your fitness level in table 3.9 opposite your age. For example, a twenty-five-year-old woman in good physical condition with a fifteen-second heart rate of 40 would have a fitness index score (from table 3.8) of 32. In table 3.9, a score of 32 opposite the age of twenty-five falls into the "average" category. Shifting one category to the right (female adjustment) gives a fitness level of "good."

Record the results of this bicycle ergometer test on your fitness evaluation form in table 3.21.

Swimming Test

The energy demands for swimming are much greater and subject to more variables than running-type exercises. Wide variations in individual skills levels directly affect energy requirements. For example, a highly skilled swimmer expends much less energy for a given distance than an individual with low-level skills. In addition to differences in swimming abilities, many individuals have difficulty breathing efficiently while swimming (mainly while doing the crawl), which can result in premature fatigue. It also is possible for an unskilled swimmer to score in the "excellent" category on the 1.5-mile run and in the "poor" category on the swimming test. Even individuals with good swimming skills who have not swam in some time may experience premature fatigue until the specific muscles needed for swimming have been properly conditioned. Therefore, the specific nature of the swimming test makes it a more appropriate test for evaluating cardiovascular fitness if you plan to participate in a swimming program.

Table 3.8 Bicycle Ergometer Fitness Index

Fifteen-second heart rate	Men: 900 kpm/min	Women: 600 kpm/min	Poorly conditioned men or men over forty: 300 kpm/min	Poorly conditioned women or women over forty: 300 kpm/min
28	75	63	32	38
29	72	61	32	37
30	70	59	31	37
31	65	55	31	35
32	60	50	30	32
33	58	47	30	29
34	55	45	26	28
35	52	41	24	26
36	49	39	22	25
37	46	38	21	24
38	45	36	20	24
39	43	33		
40	41	32		
41	39	30		
42	38	29		
43	37	28		
44	35	27		
45	34	26		

Table 3.9 Range of Maximum Oxygen Uptake (ml/kg/min) Values with Age

Age group (years)	Fitness level						
	Very poor	Poor	Average	Good	Very good	Excellent	Superior
10–19	Below 30	30–35	35–38	38–46	47–56	57–66	Above 66
20–29	Below 25	25–31	31–33	33–42	43–52	53–62	Above 62
30–39	Below 23	23–25	25–30	30–38	39–48	49–58	Above 58
40–49	Below 21	21–23	23–26	26–35	36–44	45–54	Above 54
50–59	Below 19	19–21	21–24	24–33	34–41	42–50	Above 50
60–69	Below 18	18–20	20–22	22–30	31–38	39–46	Above 46
70–79	Below 17	17–19	19–20	20–27	28–35	36–42	Above 42

Source: From Fox, E. L., Bicycle Ergometer Test, in *Journal of Applied Physiology*. Copyright 1973 American Physiological Association. Reprinted by permission.

Note: Since females are generally 20 percent lower (on average) compared to males, normal values for females can be obtained by shifting over one category to the right. For example, the "average" category for males would be considered "good" for females.

Table 3.10 Swimming Fitness

Distance in yards	Approximate time in minutes	Fitness level
700+	12 min	Superior
600–700	10–12 min	Excellent
500–600	10–12 min	Very good
400–500	10–12 min	Good
300–400	10–12 min	Average
200–300	8–10 min	Poor
0–200	6–8 min	Very poor

Source: From *The Aerobics Program for Total Well Being* by Kenneth H. Cooper, M.D., M.P.H. Copyright © 1982 by Kenneth H. Cooper. Reprinted by permission of the publisher, M. Evans & Co., Inc., 216 East 49th Street, New York, NY 10017.

The test directions are as follows:

1. Warm up a few minutes by stretching before getting into the water.
2. Start off gradually and swim until you feel fatigued (out of breath). Do not push yourself to the limit.
3. Do not swim more than twelve minutes.
4. Determine the total distance and the total time you swim.

Now find your fitness level in table 3.10. If your time falls above the time listed in the table for the distance that you completed, drop down one level to determine your score. Add fifty yards to your distance completed for each ten years over thirty years of age to arrive at an age-corrected fitness level. Record the results of this test on your fitness evaluation form in table 3.22.

Tests for Body Composition

As discussed in chapter 1, **body composition** refers to the proportion of body fat to lean body tissue. The recommended percentage of body fat for adult males is 15 percent; for adult females, 26 percent; for preadolescent boys, 5 to 8 percent; and for preadolescent girls, 10 to 11 percent.

Approximately 50 percent of the body's fat is located just below the skin. The **skinfold test** for the determination of body fat is based on the relationship of subcutaneous fat (fat just below the skin) to total lean body tissue. Unfortunately, the skinfold test is subject to error. In some cases, a 3 percent error can result when different people evaluate the same individual using skin calipers. In addition, dehydration can affect the skinfold test as much as 10 to 15 percent.

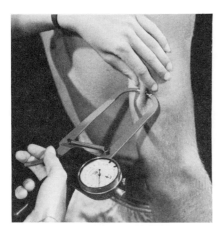

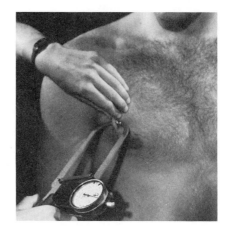

Figure 3.1 Triceps skinfold measurement. Locate a vertical skinfold on the back of the arm halfway between the tip of the acromion process (bony projection on the tip of the shoulder) and the olecranon process (rear point of the elbow), with the arm hanging in a relaxed position.

Figure 3.2 Chest skinfold measurement. Locate a point over the outside edge of the pectoralis major muscle just adjacent and medial to the armpit. The skinfold should run diagonally between the shoulder and the opposite hip.

Underwater weighing is the most accurate technique for determining body composition. However, it is somewhat complicated and requires expensive equipment. The skinfold method, even though subject to some error, is an inexpensive, rapid, and easy-to-learn method and gives you a good idea of your present percentage of body fat.

Skinfold Test

The skinfold test requires three skinfold measurements for both male and female: the chest, thigh, and abdomen for the male and the triceps, thigh, and iliac crest for the female. To perform the test, you need a pair of skinfold calipers (or you can use the pinch test described later in the chapter). Hold the skinfold between the thumb and index finger. Release the tension on the calipers slowly so that they pinch the skinfold as close as possible to your fingers. Then simply read the number from the gauge.

Figures 3.1–3.5 illustrate the methods of taking the various skinfold measurements.

After taking the three skinfold measurements appropriate for you, total the measurements. Then, on the nomogram in figure 3.6, use a ruler to connect the point on the left that corresponds to your age with the point on the far right that

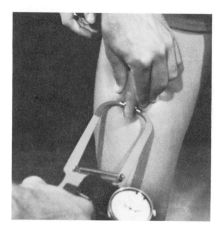

Figure 3.3 Thigh skinfold measurement. Locate a vertical skinfold in the anterior midline of the thigh, halfway between the hip and the knee joint. Place your body weight on the opposite leg while taking the measurement.

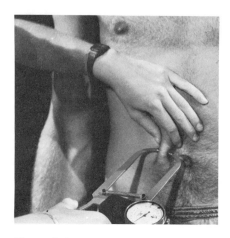

Figure 3.4 Abdomen skinfold measurement. Locate a vertical skinfold adjacent to the umbilicus.

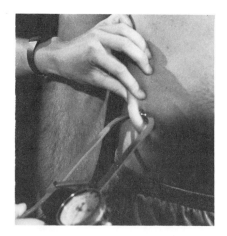

Figure 3.5 Iliac crest skinfold measurement. Locate a vertical skinfold over the iliac crest (point of the hip) in the midaxillary line (middle of the armpit).

Figure 3.6 Nomogram for the determination of percentage of body fat for the sum of the chest, abdomen, and thigh skinfolds of males fifteen years of age and above, and for the sum of the triceps, thigh, and iliac crest skinfolds of females fifteen years of age and above. (See next page.) Adapted from W. B. Baun, M. R. Baun, and P. B. Raven, "A Nomogram for the Estimate of Percent Body Fat from Generalized Equations," *Research Quarterly for Exercise and Sport* 52(1981): 380–84. Reprinted by permission of the American Alliance for Health, Physical Education, Recreation and Dance, 1900 Association Drive, Reston, Virginia 22091.

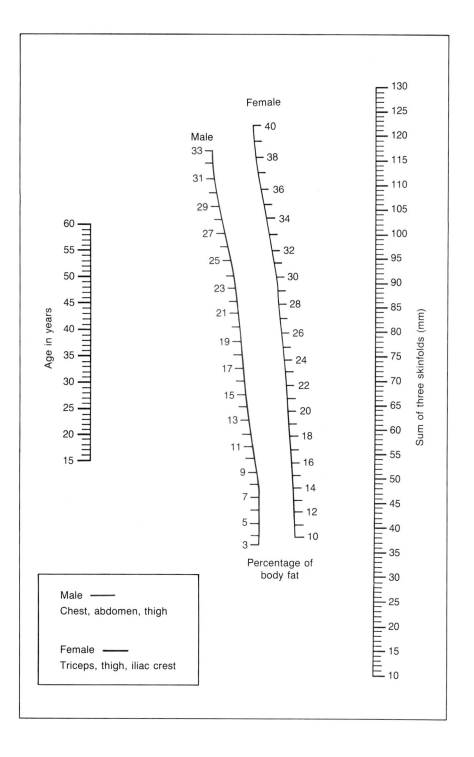

Table 3.11 Body Fat Score

Male percentage of body fat	Fitness level	Female percentage of body fat	Fitness level
Very lean	10 Superior	Very lean	13 Superior
	11–12 Excellent		13–15 Excellent
Lean	12–14 Very good	Lean	17–18 Very good
	14–15 Good		18–22 Good
Acceptable	15–17 Average	Acceptable	22–28 Average
Fat	17–18 Poor	Fat	28–30 Poor
Obese	20+ Very poor	Obese	30+ Very poor

corresponds to the sum of your three skinfold measurements. Then read the percentage of body fat from the center male or female scale. Now use your percentage of body fat to find your fitness level in table 3.11, and record the results on your fitness evaluation form (table 3.23).

Pinch Test

Pinch the skin on the back of the upper arm above the elbow and below the shoulders. Be sure not to grab muscle tissue. If the thickness of the fold is more than an inch, you may have an excess accumulation of fat. This is a rough measure but can be useful if you cannot obtain a pair of skin calipers. Record your pinch test measurement on your fitness evaluation form (table 3.24).

Tests for Flexibility

The back hyperextension test and the sit and reach test that follow are excellent measures of trunk **flexibility** (the extent and range of motion around a joint).

Back Hyperextension Test

Hyperextension involves extension of a muscle beyond its normal range. For the back hyperextension test, lie in a prone position on the floor. With your feet being held in place, arch your back and slowly and gently lift your chin and chest as far off the floor as possible (figure 3.7). The distance between the floor and the sternal notch (the groove at the top of the sternum where the clavicle attaches)

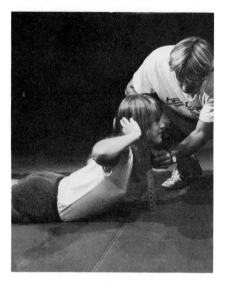

Figure 3.7 Back hyperextension test.

Table 3.12 Back Hyperextension Score

Flexibility score	Fitness level	
25 or lower	Very poor	_____
26–35	Poor	_____
36–45	Average	_____
46–50	Good	_____
51–55	Very good	_____
56–57	Excellent	_____
58+	Superior	_____

Source: Standards for Sit and Reach and Back Hyperextension, "Health Improvement Program," National Athletic Health Institute.

is measured. Then sit on the floor with your back and buttocks against a wall and measure the distance between the floor and the sternal notch (**seated sternal height**). Your flexibility score is determined by the following equation:

$$\text{Back hyperextension} = \frac{\text{Hyperextended height}}{\text{Seated sternal height}} \times 100$$

Find your score in table 3.12 and there determine your fitness level. Record your score and fitness level on your fitness evaluation form (table 3.25).

Sit and Reach Test

Sit with your legs extended directly in front of you and with the backs of your knees pressed against the floor. Your feet should be placed up against a stool to which a yardstick has been attached. The yardstick should be on top of the stool, with the fourteen-inch mark placed at the point where your foot contacts the stool. Place the index fingers of both of your hands together and reach forward as far as possible, keeping your knees in contact with the floor at all times (figure 3.8). From the yardstick, note the distance you are able to reach.

Find your score in table 3.13 and then determine your fitness level. Record your score and fitness level on your fitness evaluation form (table 3.26).

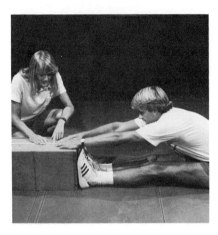

Figure 3.8 Sit and reach test.

Table 3.13 Sit and Reach Score

Sit and reach score	Fitness level	
11 in or less	Very poor	_____
12 to 13 in	Poor	_____
14 to 16 in	Average	_____
16 to 18 in	Good	_____
20 to 21 in	Very good	_____
22 to 23 in	Excellent	_____
24+ in	Superior	_____

Source: Standards for Sit and Reach and Back Hyperextension, "Health Improvement Program," National Athletic Health Institute.

Tests for Muscle Strength and Endurance

Muscle Strength Tests

Muscle strength is the amount of force that can be expected by a muscle group for one movement or repetition. It can be easily assessed by the one-repetition maximum test (1 RM)—the maximum amount of weight you can successfully lift once. Four muscle groups are tested in this section. For each, determine the greatest weight that you can lift just once for that particular lift. Begin with a weight that you can lift comfortably. Then keep adding weight until you can lift the weight correctly just one time. If you can lift the weight more than once, more pounds should be added until a true 1 RM is reached. Figures 3.9–3.12 illustrate the four lifts used to evaluate strength.

For each muscle group, divide the total amount of weight lifted by your present body weight in pounds to determine the percentage of weight lifted. Now find your percentages in table 3.14, and record your scores on your fitness evaluation form (table 3.27).

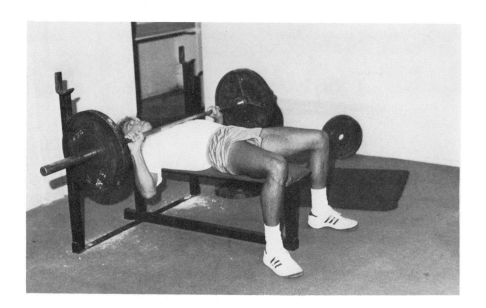

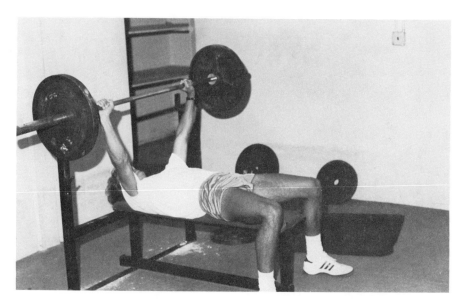

Figure 3.9 Bench press. From a supine position on a bench, take the weight with an overhand grip, hands shoulder-width apart, elbows fully extended. Lower the weight to your chest and return to your starting position. Progressively increase the weight until you can no longer make the lift.

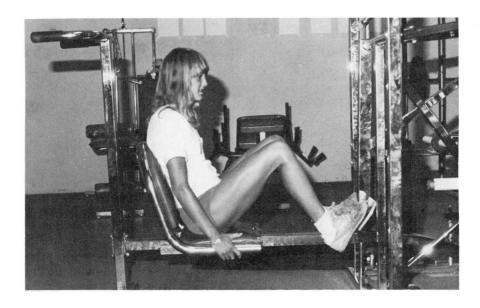

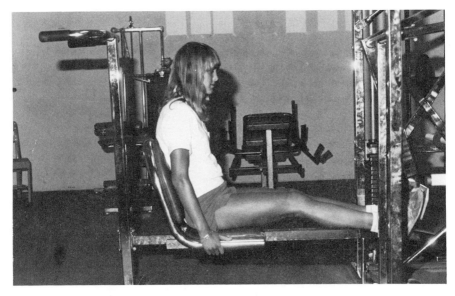

Figure 3.10 Leg press. Place your feet on the pedals and grasp the handles on the seat. Press your feet forward to elevate the weight and return. Inhale while lowering the weight and exhale while lifting it.

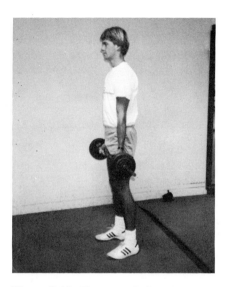

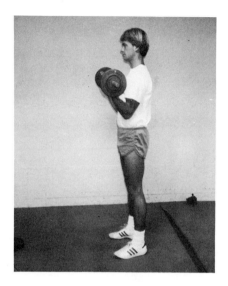

Figure 3.11 Biceps curl. Grasp the bar with your hands shoulder-width apart, using an underhand grip. Bring the bar to a position of rest against your thigh, with your elbows fully extended and your feet spread shoulder-width apart. Using only your arms, raise the bar to your chest and then return to the starting position. Keep your back straight and always return to a position where your elbows are fully extended.

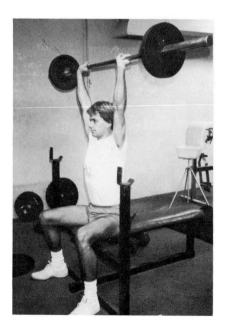

Figure 3.12 Shoulder press. Sit with your feet shoulder-width apart on the floor. Then bend your knees to forty-five degrees and grasp the bar with an overhand grip, hands spread shoulder-width apart. With your elbows under the bar, lift the weight over your head and return to your starting position.

Table 3.14 Muscle Strength Scores

		Fitness level						
Male	**Percentage of weight lifted**	**Very poor**	**Poor**	**Average**	**Good**	**Very good**	**Excellent**	**Superior**
Bench press	_____	50	75	100	110	120	140	150
Leg press	_____	160	180	200	210	220	230	240
Biceps curl	_____	30	40	50	55	60	70	80
Shoulder press	_____	40	50	67	70	80	110	120

		Fitness level						
Female	**Percentage of weight lifted**	**Very poor**	**Poor**	**Average**	**Good**	**Very good**	**Excellent**	**Superior**
Bench press	_____	40	60	70	75	80	90	100
Leg press	_____	100	120	140	145	150	175	190
Biceps curl	_____	15	20	35	40	45	55	60
Shoulder press	_____	20	30	47	55	60	60	80

Source: From *Health and Fitness through Physical Activity* by M. L. Pollock, J. H. Wilmore, and S. M. Fox. Copyright © 1978 by John Wiley & Sons. Reprinted with permission of the publisher.

Muscle Endurance Tests

Muscle endurance is to some degree dependent on your muscle strength. You may have enough strength to lift a box of groceries, but muscle endurance is necessary to hold it in your arms for the two or three minutes it takes you to move it from the store to your car. Two tests that are widely used to measure muscular endurance are push-ups (shoulder, arm, and chest muscle endurance) and sit-ups (abdominal muscle endurance).

Push-ups

Start in a standard "up" position for a full push-up, with your weight on your toes and hands. (Women can perform this test with their knees bent and their weight on their knees and hands.) Your partner should place his or her fist on the floor beneath your chest. Lower yourself down until your chest touches your

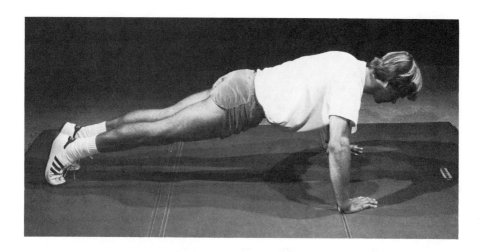

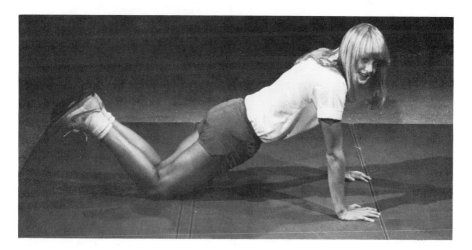

Figure 3.13 Push-ups.

partner's fist. Keep your back straight while raising to an "up" position (figure 3.13). Count the number of consecutively performed push-ups and then refer to table 3.15 to determine your fitness level. Record your score and fitness level on your fitness evaluation form (table 3.28).

Table 3.15 Push-up Muscular Endurance Test Standards

Males push-up

Age (years)	Fitness level						
	Superior	Excellent	Very good	Good	Average	Poor	Very poor
15–29	Above 51	51–54	45–50	35–44	25–34	20–25	15–19
30–39	Above 41	41–44	35–40	25–34	20–24	15–20	8–14
40–49	Above 36	35–39	30–35	20–29	14–19	12–14	5–11
50–59	Above 31	31–34	25–30	15–24	12–14	8–12	3–7
60–69	Above 26	26–29	20–25	10–19	8–9	5–7	0–4

Females modified push-up

Age (years)	Fitness level						
	Superior	Excellent	Very good	Good	Average	Poor	Very poor
15–29	Above 48	46–48	34–45	17–33	10–16	6–9	0–5
30–39	Above 38	33–37	25–33	12–24	8–11	4–7	0–3
40–49	Above 33	29–32	20–28	8–19	6–7	3–5	0–2
50–59	Above 26	21–25	15–21	6–14	4–5	2–3	0–1
60–69	Above 20	15–19	5–15	3–4	2–3	1–2	0–

Source: From *Health and Fitness through Physical Activity* by M. L. Pollock, J. H. Wilmore, and S. M. Fox. Copyright © 1978 by John Wiley & Sons. Reprinted with permission of the publisher.

Bent-Knee Sit-Ups

Even though it is difficult to measure abdominal muscle endurance, the bent-knee sit-up is the best test available. The sit-up, when performed with the knees bent, depends not only on the abdominal muscles but also the hip flexors.

Lie on your back. Cross your arms on your chest and place your hands on opposite shoulders or use an alternative position with hands clasped behind head. Your knees should be bent at about ninety degrees with both feet flat and no more than eighteen inches in front of the buttocks. Your partner should hold your feet stationary by grasping them at the ankles (figure 3.14). Complete as many sit-ups as possible in one minute. Warm up with a few sit-ups before the test.

Refer to table 3.16 to determine your fitness level. Record your score and fitness level on your fitness evaluation form (table 3.29).

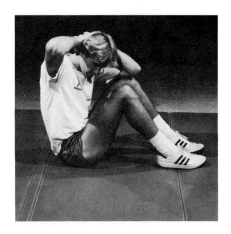

Figure 3.14 Bent-knee sit-ups.

Table 3.16 Bent-Knee Sit-ups Score

Age (years)	Very poor	Poor	Average	Good	Very good	Excellent	Superior
Fitness level							
Males							
17–29	0–17	17–35	36–41	42–47	48–50	51–55	55+
30–39*	0–13	13–26	27–32	33–38	39–43	44–48	48+
40–49	0–11	11–22	23–27	28–33	34–38	39–43	43+
50–59	0–8	8–16	17–21	22–28	29–33	34–38	38+
60–69	0–6	6–12	13–17	18–24	25–30	31–35	35+
Females							
17–29	0–14	14–28	29–32	33–35	36–42	43–47	47+
30–39*	0–11	11–22	23–28	29–34	35–40	41–45	45+
40–49	0–9	9–18	19–23	24–30	31–34	35–40	40+
50–59	0–6	6–12	13–17	18–24	25–30	31–35	35+
60–69	0–5	5–10	11–14	15–20	21–25	26–30	30+

Source: Reprinted by permission of the American Alliance for Health, Physical Education, Recreation, and Dance, 1900 Association Drive, Reston, Virginia 22091.
*The value of ages over thirty is estimated.

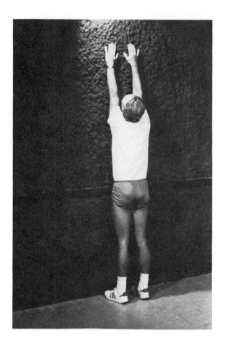 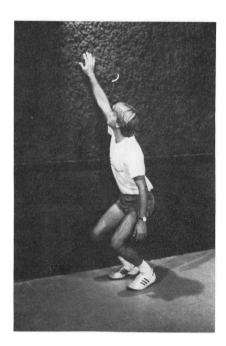

Figure 3.15 Leg power test.

Test for Leg Power

Leg power is the ability of your leg muscles to mobilize strength in a short period of time. Lower-body power is the application of strength through the dimension of time.

For the leg power test, a piece of cloth tape or a chalkboard is attached vertically to a wall. With chalked fingertips, stand facing the wall with both arms extended overhead and feet and chin touching the wall. Mark the point where your fingertips touch the tape or chalkboard. Then stand at a right angle to the taped wall. Take a deep squat position with your knees bent at forty-five degrees and your trunk bent forward thirty to forty-five degrees. Jump, touching the tape or chalkboard at the highest point that you can (figure 3.15). Record the difference between the prejump touch mark and the postjump touch mark. Then find your score in table 3.17.

Record your score and fitness level on your fitness evaluation form (table 3.30).

Table 3.17 Leg Power Score

Difference between prejump and postjump touch marks	Fitness level	
7 in	Very poor	_____
10 in	Poor	_____
16 in	Average	_____
18 in	Good	_____
20 in	Very good	_____
22 in	Excellent	_____
24+ in	Superior	_____

Determining Your Fitness Profile

Use figures 3.16 and 3.17 to determine your fitness profile. With figure 3.16, fill in the circles that correspond to your fitness level for each activity and then connect the circles with straight lines. The resulting graph shows your fitness profile. Reevaluate and rescore every six to eight weeks.

With figure 3.17, mark your predominant fitness level for each of the four basic components of physical fitness with a small circle and then connect the four circles with straight lines. The smaller and more symmetrical the square you can draw by connecting the four fitness categories, the better your overall fitness level. Fill out the paradigm every six to eight weeks to chart your progress.

Key Terms

Body Composition The proportion of body fat to lean body tissue

Cardiovascular Efficiency The ability of the heart to deliver oxygen to all of the vital organs of the body

Flexibility The extent and range of motion around a joint

Hyperextension Extension of a muscle beyond its normal range

Leg Power The ability of the leg muscles to mobilize strength in a short period of time

Muscle Strength The force produced by a muscle group

Seated Sternal Height The distance between the floor and the sternal notch while in a sitting position

Skinfold Test The method of estimating body fat by measuring subcutaneous fat with skinfold calipers

Name _____

Date _____

Fitness level	Cardiovascular					Body composition	Flexibility		Muscle strength				Muscle endurance		Leg power
	1.5-mile run	Two-minute jogging-in-place test	Step test	Bicycle ergometer test	Swimming test	Skinfold test	Back hyperextension test	Sit and reach test	Bench press test	Leg press test	Biceps curl test	Shoulder press test	Push-ups test	Bent-knee sit-ups test	Vertical jump test
Superior	o	o	o	o	o	o	o	o	o	o	o	o	o	o	o
Excellent	o	o	o	o	o	o	o	o	o	o	o	o	o	o	o
Very good	o	o	o	o	o	o	o	o	o	o	o	o	o	o	o
Good	o	o	o	o	o	o	o	o	o	o	o	o	o	o	o
Average	o	o	o	o	o	o	o	o	o	o	o	o	o	o	o
Poor	o	o	o	o	o	o	o	o	o	o	o	o	o	o	o
Very poor	o	o	o	o	o	o	o	o	o	o	o	o	o	o	o

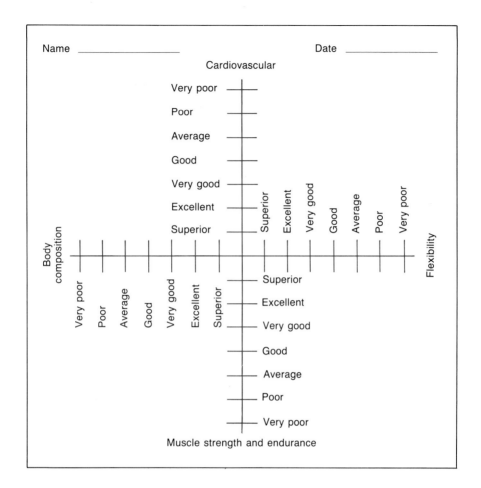

Figure 3.17 Fitness paridigm.

Figure 3.16 Fitness level and progress chart profile. (Figure on page 40.)

Physical Fitness Evaluation Form

Name _____ Age _____ Height _____ Weight _____ Sex _____

Table 3.18 1.5-Mile Run	**Table 3.19** Step Test

Time: min _____ sec _____	Resting pulse count _____
Estimated $V\dot{O}_2$ max (ml/kg/min): _____	Postexercise pulse count _____
	(per fifteen seconds)
Fitness level	Body weight _____
Very poor _____	Fitness score _____
Poor _____	Age-adjusted fitness score _____
Average _____	
Good _____	**Fitness level**
Very good _____	Very poor _____
Excellent _____	Poor _____
Superior _____	Average _____
	Good _____
Retest in six to eight weeks.	Very good _____
Date _____	Excellent _____
	Superior _____
	Retest in six to eight weeks.
	Date _____

Table 3.20 Two-Minute Jogging-in-Place Test

Preexercise thirty-second pulse rate   _____

Postexercise thirty-second pulse rate   _____

Difference between preexercise and postexercise
thirty-second pulse rate   _____

Fitness level

Very poor   _____

Poor   _____

Average   _____

Good   _____

Very good   _____

Excellent   _____

Superior   _____

Retest in six to eight weeks.   Date _____

Table 3.21 Bicycle Ergometer Test

Exercise heart rate   _____ (per minute)

Estimated $\dot{V}O_2$ max (ml/kg/min)   _____

Fitness level

Very poor   _____

Poor   _____

Average   _____

Good   _____

Very good   _____

Excellent   _____

Superior   _____

Retest in six to eight weeks.   Date _____

Table 3.22 Swimming Test

Distance swam   _____ (yards)

Approximate time _____ (minutes)

Fitness level

Very poor

Poor   _____

Average   _____

Good   _____

Very good   _____

Excellent   _____

Superior   _____

Retest in six to eight weeks.   Date _____

Table 3.23 Skinfold Test

Male: Chest _____ Abdomen _____ Thigh _____ Total _____

Female: Triceps _____ Iliac crest _____ Thigh _____ Total _____

Percentage of body fat _____

Fitness level

Very poor   _____

Poor   _____

Average   _____

Good   _____

Very good   _____

Excellent   _____

Superior   _____

Retest in six to eight weeks.   Date _____

Table 3.24 Pinch Test

Measurement of skinfold _____ inches

Retest in six to eight weeks.
Date _____

Table 3.25 Back Hyperextension Test

Hyperextended height   _____

Seated sternal height   _____

Flexibility score   _____

Fitness level

Very poor   _____

Poor   _____

Average   _____

Good   _____

Very good   _____

Excellent   _____

Superior   _____

Retest in six to eight weeks.
Date _____

Table 3.26 Sit and Reach Test

Sit and reach score _____

Fitness level

Very poor   _____

Poor   _____

Average   _____

Good   _____

Very good   _____

Excellent   _____

Superior   _____

Retest in six to eight weeks.   Date _____

Table 3.27 Muscle Strength Tests

Male	Percentage of weight lifted	Very poor	Poor	Average	Good	Very good	Excellent	Superior
		Fitness level						
Bench press	_____	50	75	100	110	120	140	150
Leg press	_____	160	180	200	210	220	230	240
Biceps curl	_____	30	40	50	55	60	70	80
Shoulder press	_____	40	50	67	70	80	110	120

Female	Percentage of weight lifted	Very poor	Poor	Average	Good	Very good	Excellent	Superior
		Fitness level						
Bench press	_____	40	60	70	75	80	90	100
Leg press	_____	100	120	140	145	150	175	190
Biceps curl	_____	15	20	35	40	45	55	60
Shoulder press	_____	20	30	47	55	60	60	80

Retest in six to eight weeks.   Date _____

Table 3.28 Push-ups Test

Number of push-ups _____

Fitness level

Very poor _____

Poor _____

Average _____

Good _____

Very good _____

Excellent _____

Superior _____

Retest in six to eight weeks.

Date _____

Table 3.29 Bent-Knee Sit-ups Test

Number of sit-ups _____

Fitness level

Very poor _____

Poor _____

Average _____

Good _____

Very good _____

Excellent _____

Superior _____

Retest in six to eight weeks.

Date _____

Table 3.30 Leg Power Test

Difference between prejump and postjump touch marks _____

Fitness level

Very poor _____

Poor _____

Average _____

Good _____

Very good _____

Excellent _____

Superior _____

Retest in six to eight weeks.   Date _____

Warm-up and Flexibility

Warm-up and Exercise

The term **warm-up** has a variety of meanings. To one person, it may mean a few push-ups and jumping jacks; to another, it may mean stretching and flexibility exercises; to someone else, it may mean jogging for fifteen or twenty minutes. Regardless of what they actually entail, there is general agreement that warm-up exercises are essential to prepare the heart, lungs, and muscles to adequately meet the subsequent demands placed on them during rigorous physical exercise and that they are an important prerequisite to all physical activity.

Generally, there are three types of warm-up exercises. The first is a type of specific neuromuscular warm-up where the skill is performed at a less intense level prior to the actual activity to ensure that the proper muscles are being stimulated and that the coordination and skill level are maximized. In other words, the type of warm-up is specific to the type of activity that is to follow. For example, hurdlers generally do not do push-ups before a race but engage in some mild running and practice the specific leg movement involved in hurdling. Many athletes believe that this type of warm-up must precede an activity to produce optimal skilled performance.

The second type of warm-up exercises involves using static stretching techniques to stretch the muscles prior to an activity. Stretching increases extensibility and reduces the resistance of the muscles. It also produces more efficient muscle contractions and reduces the chances of injury or soreness.

The third type of warm-up exercises is concerned with general body warm-up. The exercises, such as jogging or calisthenics, are aimed at increasing the body temperature and gradually stimulating the heart. Substantial evidence indicates that, when the body temperature is increased at least one degree Fahrenheit, a number of changes that aid physical performance occur in the muscles and circulatory system. General body warm-up also prepares the heart to meet efficiently the stressful demands placed upon it during vigorous exercise and helps to prevent the possibility of heart damage during the initial stages of exercise. Recent research has shown abnormalities in electrocardiograms of individuals who did not warm up prior to exercise. It is therefore vital to gradually stimulate the cardiovascular system with a general warm-up activity before engaging in rigorous exercise. Subjecting the heart to a sudden overload without a warm-up can result in a reduced flow of blood to the heart muscles, which could lead to serious consequences.

Flexibility

Flexibility is generally defined as a looseness or suppleness of the joint. More specifically, flexibility is the range and the extent of the movement of a joint. Some individuals have a wide range of motion; others' range of motion is fairly limited.

Joint flexibility is controlled by a number of factors: the joint capsule contributes approximately 47 percent to the range of motion, the muscles contribute 41 percent, the tendons contribute 10 percent, and the skin contributes 2 percent. Because the joint capsule itself is rigid, the emphasis when attempting to increase or decrease flexibility is placed on the muscle and skin tissue. Stretching exercises enable these tissues to increase the range of the movement. Conversely, strengthening exercises tighten up the muscles and tendons and can decrease the range of movement.

Women tend to have a greater range of movement in the joints than men primarily because men have generally larger and bulkier skeletal muscles, which tend to reduce joint movement. However, flexibility from individual to individual varies widely.

All activities require varying degrees of flexibility. A competitive tennis player needs good shoulder flexibility. A laborer requires good lower-back flexibility. Even such everyday movements as walking and running require flexibility. Good flexibility reduces the possibility of the aches, pains, and inflammations associated with joints that are stressed through rigorous activity.

The Importance of Stretching

Stretching involves extending and holding muscles for a specific period of time to increase range of movement in a joint. Failure to stretch muscle tissue regularly can lead to a decrease in soft tissue elasticity.

Two kinds of stretching exercises—static and ballistic—increase flexibility. **Static stretching** consists of stretching the muscle slowly and gradually for periods of six to ten seconds, followed by several seconds of relaxation. This method is a very effective stretching technique and does not impose unnecessary stress on the muscle. **Ballistic stretching,** on the other hand, involves rapid bouncing, jerking movements, which have the potential for injuring soft muscle and joint tissue. The ballistic method of jerking and bouncing actually invokes what is called a stretch reflex, which opposes the desired stretching and can result in muscle soreness. Ballistic stretching is not recommended.

Key Warm-up Principles

1. No matter what the nature of the exercise to come, a slow, gradual warm-up, consisting of calisthenics, stretching, and slow jogging, always should precede exercise, even if you are highly trained.
2. Be ready to make minor adjustments to your stretching routine. You may be more flexible on some days than others.
3. Your warm-up should last ten to fifteen minutes.
4. Initial stretching should be gentle and specific to the muscles that will receive the most stress.
5. Jogging should be conducted at an intensity and rate specific to your anticipated activity and level of fitness.
6. Stretching following mild jogging should be slow but thorough.
7. Only a few minutes should lapse between the completion of the warm-up and the activity.
8. Experiment with different types of warm-ups. Find the one that best fits your body. The warm-up should feel good.
9. A portion of the warm-up exercise should consist of skill drills and other skilled movements related to the anticipated activity to follow the warm-up.

Stretching Exercises

The stretching exercises illustrated and explained in figures 4.1–4.7 include all of the major muscle groups in the body and thus are preparatory for the majority of physical activities in which you might wish to participate. Use record sheets B-1 and B-2 in Appendix B at the back of the book to record your progress with these exercises.

The "Easy Seven"

Cyclists, runners, and swimmers should engage in other special stretching exercises, in addition to the "Easy Seven" stretching exercises shown in figures 4.1–4.7. Special stretching exercises for cyclists are illustrated and explained in figures 4.8–4.11; figures 4.12–4.15 show stretching exercises for runners; and swimmers' stretching exercises are demonstrated in figures 4.16–4.21.

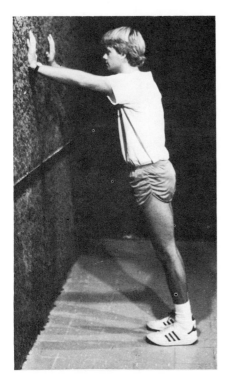

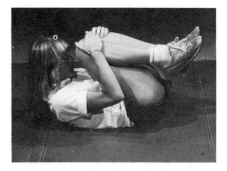

Figure 4.2 Back stretch. While lying on your back, bring both of your knees to your chest. Grasp both of your legs below the knees and pull the knees toward your chest. Hold for ten seconds. Repeat ten times.

Figure 4.1 Achilles tendon stretch. (The **Achilles tendon** is a large tendon connecting the calf muscle to the heel.) Face a wall and stand approximately three feet in front of it with your feet several inches apart. Place your outstretched hands on the wall while keeping your feet flat on the floor. Gradually lean forward toward the wall. Hold the stretch for ten seconds. Repeat five times.

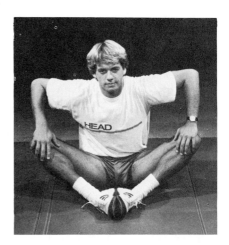

Figure 4.3 Groin stretch. Sit on the floor with the soles of your feet touching in front of you. Gradually push your knees down as far as possible. Hold the final stretched position for five seconds. Repeat five times. Each day try to push your knees closer to the floor.

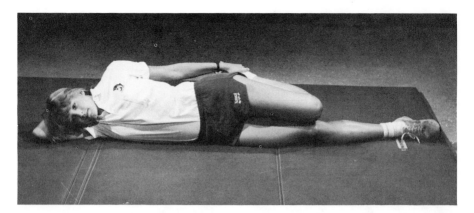

Figure 4.4 Quadriceps stretch. While lying on your left side, flex the knee of your right leg and grab the ankle with your right hand. Gradually move your hip forward until a good stretch is felt on the thigh. Hold for five seconds. Repeat five times. Repeat for the left leg while lying on your right side.

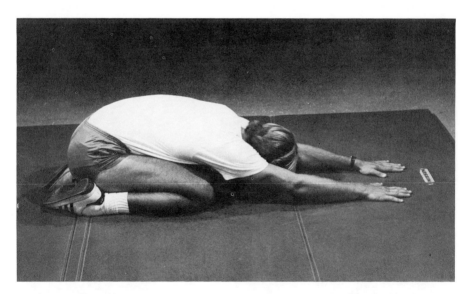

Figure 4.5 Abdominal stretch. Get down on all fours by placing your hands and knees on the floor. Lean back onto your heels. Extend your arms and place your chest on the floor. Hold for ten seconds. Repeat five times.

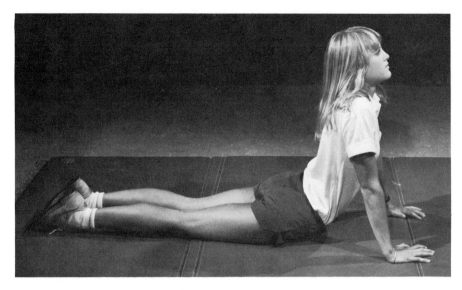

Figure 4.6 Upper-trunk stretch. While lying on your stomach, push your upper body off the mat to a position where your arms are fully extended. Try to keep your hips and pelvis on the floor. Hold for ten seconds. Repeat five times.

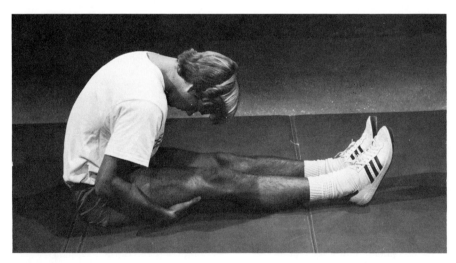

Figure 4.7 Lower-back stretch. While sitting on the floor with your legs extended out in front of you, force your knees flat against the floor. Grab behind your knees and slowly pull your head down toward your knees. Move slowly. Hold for ten seconds. Repeat five times.

Stretching Exercises for Cyclists

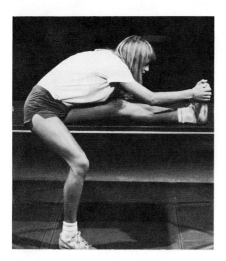

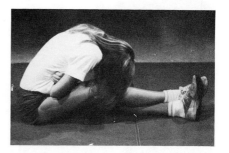

Figure 4.9 Back extensor. Sit with your legs crossed and your arms folded in front of you. Tuck your chin to your chest. Roll forward and attempt to touch your forehead to your knees. Roll forward gradually, keeping your hips on the floor. Do not bob. Hold for eight seconds. Repeat five times.

Figure 4.8 Hamstring stretch. (The **hamstring** is a group of muscles in the upper leg that are important in knee flexion.) Sit on a table with one leg extended across the table and the opposite leg hanging over the side of the table. Bend forward at the waist and reach toward the toes of your extended leg. Try to keep the leg straight. Reach gradually; do not bob. Hold for eight seconds. Repeat five times for each leg.

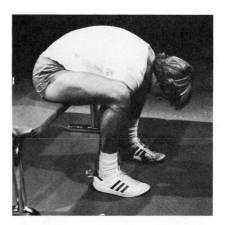

Figure 4.10 Lower-back extensor. Sit on a chair or bench with your feet flat on the floor and about six inches apart. Tuck in your chin and curl forward between your knees with your arms hanging toward the floor until you feel resistance in your back. Hold for ten seconds. Repeat five times.

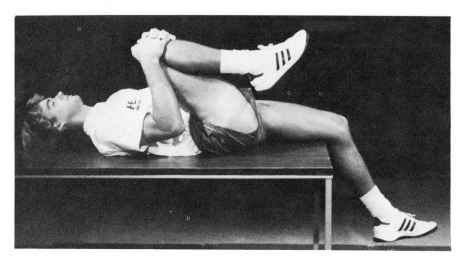

Figure 4.11 Hip flexor. Lie on your back on a table with your legs over the edge of the table. Bring your right knee to your chest. Use both of your hands on your kneecap to gradually press the knee toward your armpit. Hold for ten seconds. Repeat five times for each leg.

Stretching Exercises for Runners

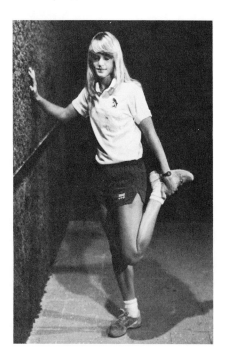

Figure 4.12 Front-leg stretch. Lean against a wall. Bring your right foot up behind you. Grasp the foot with your right hand and touch the foot to your buttocks. Hold for six seconds. Repeat five times for each leg.

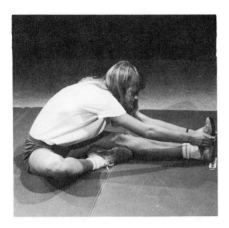

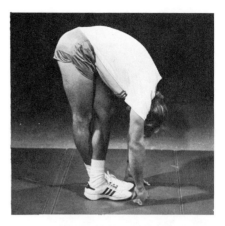

Figure 4.13 Modified hurdler stretch. Sit with your right leg extended and your left leg crossed in front with the heel near your crotch. Reach forward with your right arm as far as possible. Hold for six seconds. Repeat five times for each leg.

Figure 4.14 Standing hamstring stretch. While standing, cross one leg over the other. The toes of the front leg should just touch the floor, with your heel in the air. Bend forward from the waist while keeping the rear leg straight. Stretch until you feel resistance. Hold for six seconds. Repeat five times for each leg.

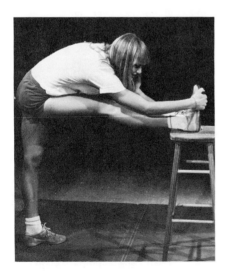

Figure 4.15 Leaning hamstring stretch. While standing, raise one leg with the toes pointing up, and rest the heel of your foot on a solid object, for example, a car bumper or bench. Lean forward and reach with both arms toward raised foot. Hold for six seconds. Repeat five times for each leg.

Stretching Exercises for Swimmers

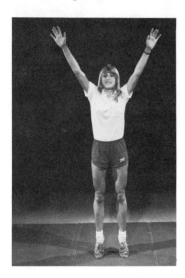

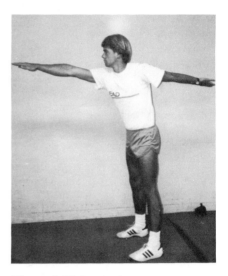

Figure 4.16 Arm and Achilles stretch. Stand with your feet shoulder-width apart. Raise your extended arms overhead. Place your weight on your toes and stretch to the sky. Hold for six seconds. Repeat five times.

Figure 4.17 Forward- and back-arm stretch. Stand with your feet shoulder-width apart. Bend forward about twenty degrees from the waist. Extend your left arm to the front and your right arm to the rear. Hold your arms shoulder high for six seconds. Repeat five times. Then reverse arm positions and repeat five times.

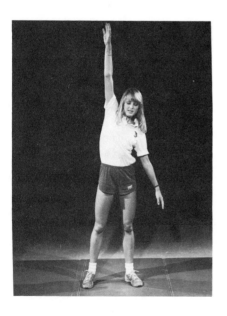

Figure 4.18 High-low arm stretch. Stand with your feet shoulder-width apart. Extend your right arm straight up from your body and extend your left arm straight down. Hold the stretch for six seconds. Repeat five times. Then reverse arm positions and repeat five times.

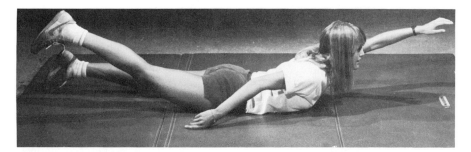

Figure 4.19 Arm and leg stretch. Lie facedown with your arms extended above your head. Slowly raise your right arm and left leg simultaneously. Hold for six seconds. Repeat five times for each side of body.

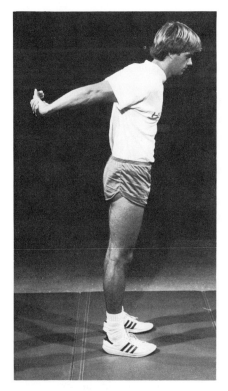

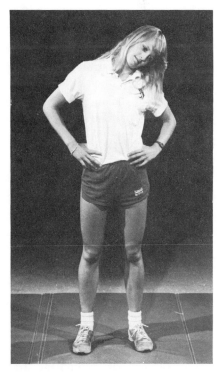

Figure 4.20 Upper-chest stretch. Stand with your feet slightly apart. Grasp your hands behind your back and raise your arms. Hold for six seconds. Repeat five times.

Figure 4.21 Neck stretch. Stand with your hands on your hips. Flex your head toward your right shoulder. Hold for six seconds. Then flex your head toward your left shoulder and hold for six seconds. Repeat five times.

Lower-Back Problems

Difficulty in straightening up after bending over, stiffness, or mild to crippling pain are common symptoms of lower-back problems. Generally, lower-back problems result from injury to muscles, ligaments, or discs in the lumbar area of the spine. Injuries to these areas are more common when the following factors are present: weak abdominal and back muscles, poor flexibility, a sedentary lifestyle, and improper sitting or lifting. Weak abdominal muscles lead to hyperextension (increasing the arch of the lower back), which puts added strain on muscles, ligaments, and spinal discs. Acute back strain that does not receive proper treatment can develop into chronic back strain.

Exercises to stretch the spine and enhance the condition of abdominal muscles are essential for prevention and rehabilitation of lower-back problems. Lower-back problems also may be prevented through observance of the following principles:

1. Maintain the strength of your abdominal muscles with conditioning exercises. Bent-knee sit-ups (see figure 3.14) are excellent abdominal strengtheners.
2. Engage in stretching exercises for the hamstrings, which aid in the prevention of lower-back problems.
3. Avoid standing for long periods of time. This can aggravate the lower back. If you must stand, shift your weight from one leg to the other and flex one knee so that one leg is supported higher than the other.
4. When lifting, keep your back straight. Lift with your leg muscles, not with your back muscles. Don't bend over without bending your knees, and keep the weight you are lifting close to your body. Avoid lifting objects above your waist, which can increase pressure on lower-back muscles and ligaments.
5. Sleep on your side with your knees bent. Do not sleep on your stomach or lie on your back with your legs straight. If you must lie on your back, bend your knees.
6. Before getting out of bed in the morning, perform a few lower-back exercises, such as single-leg or double-leg pulls (see figures 4.24 and 4.25). Then stand up slowly after leaving the bed.
7. When sitting, try to keep your knees above your hips to reduce lower-back arching and strain.
8. When kneeling down (as when doing gardening), avoid sudden lateral or turning movements with your upper body.

The exercises illustrated and explained in figures 4.22–4.25 are beneficial in the prevention and rehabilitation of lower-back pain.

Lower-Back Exercises

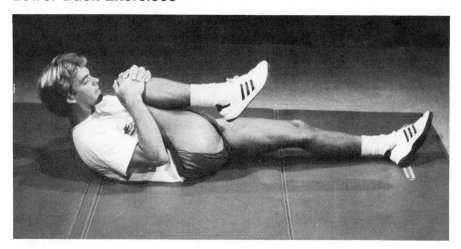

Figure 4.22 Lower-back stretch. Lie on your back with both legs straight. Bring one knee to your chest. Grasp your leg just below the knee with both hands and pull your knee toward your chest. Hold for eight to ten seconds. Then, while still grasping the knee, bring your head and shoulders toward the knee. Hold for five to eight seconds. Return to the original position and repeat the exercise using the other leg. Repeat five times.

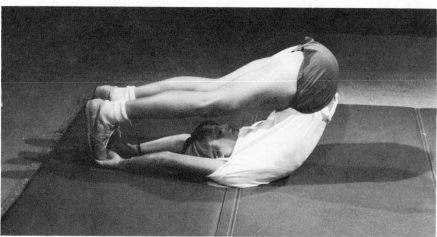

Figure 4.23 Back and leg stretch. Lie on your back. Keep both arms extended. An alternative position, keeping both hands flat on the floor by your side may also be used. Extend both of your legs over your head and try and touch your toes to the floor. Hold for eight to ten seconds. Repeat five times.

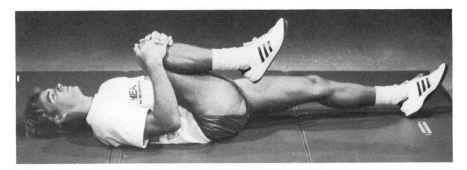

Figure 4.24 Single-leg pull. Lie on your back with both legs straight. Grasp one leg just below the knee and pull the knee to your chest. Hold for eight to ten seconds. Then alternate with the other leg. Repeat five times.

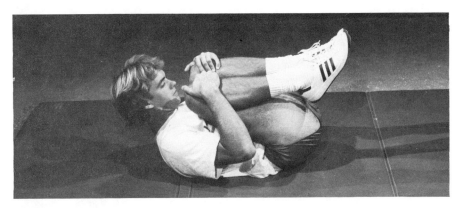

Figure 4.25 Double-leg pull. Lie on your back with both knees bent. Grasp both legs just below the knees and pull the knees to your chest. Hold for eight to ten seconds. Repeat five times.

Key Terms

Achilles Tendon A large tendon connecting the calf muscle to the heel

Ballistic Stretching Rapid bouncing, jerking types of muscle movements

Flexibility The range and the extent of the movement of a joint

Hamstring A group of muscles in the upper leg that are important in knee flexion

Static Stretching- A stretching method that consists of stretching the muscle slowly and gradually

Warm-Up Exercises performed immediately before physical activity to prepare the heart, lungs, and muscles to adequately meet the demands of rigorous exercise

Cardiovascular Fitness

The Heart

Recently, considerable research has dealt with the heart and its response to training through exercise. The relationship between exercise and coronary artery disease, which plagues thousands of individuals every year, also is being intensively investigated. There is no question that the cardiovascular system is the cornerstone of health-related fitness. A basic understanding of the heart is important for those planning to or actually engaging in physical exercise.

Structure and Function

The heart weighs less than a pound and is about the size of your fist. This powerful, long-working organ pumps blood through the blood vessels in a closed cycle within the body. The heart begins beating early in embryonic life and continues until death. During an average lifetime of sixty-five to seventy years, the heart pumps approximately 150 to 200 million liters of blood.

The human heart has four chambers (figure 5.1). The two upper chambers, where the veins empty, are called atrias, and the two lower chambers, where the blood leaves the heart, are called ventricles. The muscle walls of the atrias are very thin because, aided by gravity, they only have to pump blood into the ventricles. The ventricles, however, have to pump blood to all parts of the body, a more demanding function that requires a much larger muscle.

Blood circulates through the body in a closed cycle. "Used" blood that has given up a large portion of its oxygen and that contains high levels of carbon dioxide is returned to the heart via two large veins—the superior vena cava, which brings blood from the head, arms, and shoulders, and the inferior vena cava, which drains blood from the rest of the body below the heart—into the right

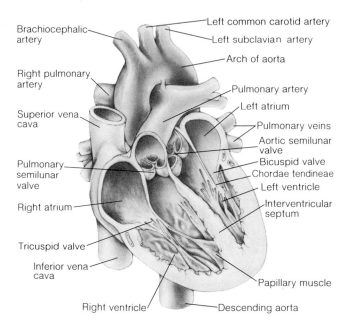

Brachiocephalic artery
Left common carotid artery
Left subclavian artery
Arch of aorta
Right pulmonary artery
Pulmonary artery
Left atrium
Superior vena cava
Pulmonary veins
Aortic semilunar valve
Bicuspid valve
Pulmonary semilunar valve
Chordae tendineae
Left ventricle
Right atrium
Interventricular septum
Tricuspid valve
Inferior vena cava
Papillary muscle
Right ventricle
Descending aorta

Figure 5.1 Anterior internal view of heart. From Van De Graaff, Kent M., *Human Anatomy Laboratory Textbook,* 2d ed. © 1981, 1984 Wm. C. Brown Publisher, Dubuque, Iowa. All rights reserved. Reprinted by permission.

atrium. From here, the blood passes through the tricuspid valve into the right ventricle. From the right ventricle, the blood leaves the heart through the pulmonary valve into the pulmonary artery, which travels to the lungs. In the lungs, the blood gives up carbon dioxide and picks up more oxygen. Two pulmonary veins from each lung carry fresh blood back to the left atrium of the heart. From the left atrium, the blood passes through the bicuspid valve into the left ventricle. From the left ventricle, the blood flows through the aortic valve into the aorta, which branches to all parts of the body. Microscopic vessels called capillaries connect the small arteries to the veins. Within the capillaries, oxygen from the blood is transferred to the cells. All of the veins eventually join the superior and inferior vena cava, which lead back to the heart, thus completing the cycle.

The sounds that you hear from a beating heart are caused by the opening and closing of the valves between the chambers of the heart and the valves in the two large arteries leaving the heart.

Maximum Oxygen Uptake and Stroke Volume

The main function of the heart and circulatory system is to provide blood, which is necessary to maintain the proper functioning of all body cells. In terms of exercise, the heart's main concern is its ability to deliver oxygen to the working cells of the body and to rid the cells of waste products. The greatest amount of oxygen utilized by the cells during maximum exercise per unit of time is referred to as **maximum oxygen uptake.** Maximum oxygen uptake is one of the best indices of cardiovascular fitness. Training may be a 20 percent contributing factor in determining maximum oxygen uptake, whereas the remaining 80 percent is thought to be genetically determined.

The amount of blood pumped out per beat (**stroke volume**) at rest for the average individual is approximately 70 to 90 milliliters. During rigorous activity, the average heart may pump 100 to 120 milliliters per beat. The trained individual, however, may have a stroke volume at rest of 100 to 120 milliliters and a maximum capability during exercise of 150 to 170 milliliters. This gives the trained individual a decided advantage since the more efficient your heart, the greater its ability to maintain exercise levels for long periods of time with less stress. The hearts of some trained individuals may be capable of pumping out as much as 30 to 35 *liters* a minute. This amount is six times the total volume of the blood in the body, which indicates the truly exceptional efficiency of the heart.

Irregular Heartbeats

Irregular heartbeats (**cardiac arrhythmia**) are considered abnormal but not necessarily dangerous. Any type of abnormal beating of the heart, however, should be carefully evaluated by a physician to determine its origin. Extra heartbeats may be caused by caffeine (found in coffee, tea, and chocolate), anxiety, or heart disease. When there is an extra heartbeat, usually one of the lower chambers of the heart (the ventricle) does not have enough time to fill with blood. As a result, a reduced amount of blood is pumped out, resulting in lowered blood pressure and producing a feeling of faintness or weakness.

Heart Murmurs

As blood passes through the heart, it makes a very distinctive noise, called a heart murmur. Some types of heart murmurs may indicate leakage of a valve. Other murmurs, sometimes found in endurance athletes, result from a stronger contraction of the heart muscle and are not important. Valvular leakage or insufficiency are common heart ailments often present in childhood, but they usually disappear as the child grows older. The seriousness of the effects on the body depends upon the valves affected or the degree of defect. It is possible to have a slight heart murmur and still engage in physical exercise, but the intensity and duration of the exercise should be determined in consultation with a physician.

Heart Rate

Normal resting heart rates may range from a low of thirty-five beats per minute to a high of one hundred beats per minute. The average for a young adult is around seventy beats per minute. Sedentary individuals usually have higher resting heart rates than physically active individuals. Individuals in excellent cardio-vascular condition generally have very low resting heart rates. This probably is due to increased efficiency of the heart muscle and changes in the nervous system. Because their hearts have a larger stroke volume, these people are able to deliver the required oxygen to their body cells at a lower heart rate. In addition, after rigorous exercise, the well-conditioned individual's heart generally returns to resting levels faster than the heart of a sedentary person.

Other factors also may play an important role in lowering resting heart rate. One finding that supports this contention is that some well-conditioned athletes have been found to have heart rates in the seventies and eighties, whereas we would expect their resting heart rates to be in the forties and fifties.

Measuring Heart Rate

In measuring heart rate, the pulse may be taken either by placing a hand directly over the heart (left breast) or by palpating the radial artery at the base of the thumb (palm side of the wrist) or the temporal artery in front of the ear. Taking the pulse at the carotid artery in the neck is not recommended since the pressure from palpating may slow the heart or cause a cardiac abnormality.

Determining the Training Effect

The proper intensity level of an endurance training program is approximately 70 percent of your maximum heart rate. This is referred to as the threshold effect or **training effect.** To determine the training effect for your heart, it is first nec-essary to determine your maximum heart rate. The direct method of exercising an individual to exhaustion on a treadmill and monitoring heart rate to determine maximum level is difficult and, for some individuals, dangerous. However, a rea-sonable estimate of your maximum heart rate can be determined by subtracting your age from 220. For example, a twenty-year-old would have a maximum heart rate of 200 (220 − 20).

The next step in determining your training effect level is to find your resting heart rate by taking your pulse for one minute shortly after you rise in the morning. To arrive at a more reliable measure, take your pulse three mornings in a row and find the average.

Next, subtract your resting heart rate from your maximum heart rate and multiply the difference by 70 percent. Add this product to your resting heart rate, which will give you your training effect level.

The following is an example of determining the training effect level for a twenty-year-old individual with a resting heart rate of eighty beats per minute:

220 − 20 = 200 beats per minute (maximum heart rate)
200 − 80 = 120 (80 is the resting heart rate in this example)
120 × .70 = 84 (.70 is the desired intensity of activity)
84 + 80 = 164 beats per minute
The training effect level in this example is 164 beats per minute.

The Ten-Second Rate

A convenient technique for counting the heart rate during exercise is determining the ten-second rate. Divide your training effect level by six, since there are six ten-second intervals in one minute. For example, an individual with a training effect level of 164 would have a ten-second heart rate of 164 ÷ 6 = approximately 27. With this method, you take your heart rate for only ten seconds, rather than having to count for an entire minute.

Perceived Exertion

It is extremely difficult to get an accurate pulse rate while exercising. In addition, when you stop exercising, your heart rate drops very rapidly, giving you an unreliable reading. Therefore, it is necessary to locate your pulse quickly to determine what level of intensity you have reached during exercise. However, once you are comfortable with your training program, you may want to experiment with an indirect technique of determining heart rate that comes pretty close to actual heart rate. This method is referred to as **perceived exertion.**

Considerable evidence indicates that normal individuals (those with an absence of neurosis or extremely high levels of anxiety) are capable of integrating various body sensations, such as body temperature, breathing intensity, muscle and joint sensations, and heart rate, to arrive at a subjective estimate of exercise intensity that approximates the actual metabolic cost of exercise.

Borg has developed a model that correlates heart rate with perceived exertion (see table 5.1). The model rates perceived exertion on a scale of 6 to 20. Multiplying the perceived exertion factor by a factor of 10 corresponds to actual heart rate at that perceived intensity level. For example, if your work intensity is perceived at an intensity of 17, the predicted heart rate would be 170 (17 × 10 = 170).

When you first begin your exercise program, you may want to use Borg's model to determine your perceived level of exercise. At various times in your exercise program, monitor your intensity level by choosing a number that you think approximates your level of exertion. When rating your perceived exertion, use a combination of all sensations of physical stress, effort, fatigue, and breathing. Don't concentrate on just one sensation, such as shortness of breath or sore leg muscles.

Table 5.1 Perceived Exertion Scale	
6	60 beats per minute
7—Very, very light	
8	
9—Very light	
10	
11—Fairly light	
12	
13—Somewhat hard	
14	
15—Hard	
16	
17—Very hard	
18	
19—Very, very hard	
20	200 beats per minute

Source: From Borg, G. A. V., "Perceived Exertion: Note on History and Method," in *Medicine & Science in Sports*, 5:90. © 1973 American College of Sports Medicine. Reprinted by permission.

Once you have decided on a level of exertion, take your heart rate for one minute. Then compare your actual heart rate with the heart rate in table 5.1 that corresponds with the number you have chosen as your perceived exertion level. With a little practice, you will be amazed how accurate you can be in predicting your heart rate. Borg's model has been found to be approximately 80 percent accurate.

This ability to predict your perceived exertion enables you to monitor your exercise and prevent excess stress and assures you of a safe exercise routine.

Anaerobic and Aerobic Exercise

All-out exercise lasting one to two minutes is referred to as **anaerobic** (without oxygen). Such exercises as weight lifting, sprinting, tennis, handball, squash, volleyball, and racquetball train the anaerobic system. Continuous rigorous exercise lasting beyond one to two minutes, such as jogging, long-distance swimming, cycling, and cross-country skiing, trains the **aerobic** system (with oxygen).

The physical demands of the all-out burst of muscle effort in anaerobic exercise require that the heart and the circulatory system be in a high state of fitness. Anaerobic activities often are competitive and may produce overexertion. Thus, even young individuals in good health should be careful not to engage in anaerobic activities until they are aerobically fit and have participated in an aerobic exercise program for several weeks. In general, if your primary concern is maintaining good cardiovascular fitness and you are not interested in competitive activities, anaerobic kinds of training can be eliminated from your exercise program with little effect on cardiovascular endurance.

Before Exercise

Before starting your cardiovascular program, you must be aware of three principles: intensity, duration, and frequency. **Intensity** refers to the degree of overload or "stressfulness" of the exercise; **duration** is the amount of time utilized for each exercise bout; and **frequency** is the number of exercise bouts per week. Generally, the more intensive, the longer, and the more frequent the training program, the greater the cardiovascular benefits.

A preexercise medical evaluation also is advised prior to beginning a cardiovascular exercise program. What time of the day would be best for your exercise and exercise precautions are two additional topics you should consider. All of these areas are explored in further detail in the sections that follow.

Intensity

For a training effect to occur within the cardiovascular and muscle systems, the exercise program must consist of activities that produce an overload on these systems. As discussed previously, research has shown that the intensity for cardiovascular training should be at 70 percent of the maximum heart rate reserve and that this training effect level must be maintained throughout the exercise period. However, low-intensity programs below the 70 percent level are appropriate for nonactive individuals who are just beginning an exercise program or those interested only in maintaining proper body weight.

Your desired exercise intensity must be gauged to your age and relative fitness. An exercise pulse rate of from 110 to 120 beats per minute for middle-aged individuals may be an effective training stimulus, whereas younger people may have to work at a steady pulse rate of from 140 to 160 beats per minute.

Duration

How long you exercise depends primarily on the intensity of the exercise and your long-range goals. Beginners should exercise for a minimum of fifteen to twenty minutes. As fitness level improves, the exercise session can be increased to thirty minutes. Maintaining your target training effect level during the thirty minutes of exercise will improve your cardiovascular fitness. Longer work periods are only necessary for those interested in competing in such activities as long-distance running or swimming. Strength training should be approximately fifteen minutes in duration.

Frequency

You don't have to knock yourself out seven days a week to achieve cardiovascular fitness. Workouts three to five days a week are sufficient. It is important to allow yourself twenty-four to forty-eight hours for rest and recovery between exercise bouts.

Overstressing the body is one of the worst things you can do, and one way to do that is by strenuously exercising only once a week. This kind of regimen is worse than no exercise at all. Strenuous exercising once a week can greatly stress your cardiovascular system without producing any benefits. If you cannot exercise at least three times a week, then your once- or twice-a-week exercise should be moderate, with the main objectives of relaxation and burning up a few extra calories.

Another thing to keep in mind is that if you miss a day or two in your exercise routine, you should never try to make it up. This is a dangerous practice, especially for middle-aged people. The important consideration here is not to become obsessive about exercising. Some people, whose main goal in exercising is to avoid having a heart attack, become so rigidly goal-directed that any interference in their exercise schedule results in anxiety. This is not the object of exercise. Your exercise program should be enjoyable and relaxing. Avoid rigidly structured schedules that lead to anxiety and tension. And remember, don't "pile it on" if you miss a day.

Preexercise Medical Evaluation

There is considerable controversy about whether a stress test is necessary before an individual begins a rigorous exercise program. The basic rationale for the stress test is that, when the heart is overloaded, as during a stress test, any abnormality present comes to light. Many abnormalities of the heart do not show up while a person is at rest—the heart needs to be under stress for them to be detected. Some individuals, however, do not show any abnormalities during a stress test and yet may have heart disease.

A generally accepted principle is that persons under thirty-five who have good medical histories usually do not need a stress test before beginning a rigorous exercise program. However, they should begin gradually if they have been leading sedentary lives. Individuals over thirty-five and especially those who have coronary risk factors, such as high blood pressure, diabetes, excess weight, a heavy smoking habit, or a family history of heart disease, should always check with a physician before starting a rigorous exercise program to ensure that there are no health problems that could be aggravated by rigorous exercise.

When to Exercise

Some individuals experience light-headedness and nausea if they exercise rigorously early in the morning before breakfast. Because they haven't had anything to eat for a number of hours, their blood sugar levels probably are low, which is the probable explanation for their discomfort. Rigorous exercise too soon after breakfast also can cause physical distress, such as a feeling of fullness or nausea. Mild stretching and calisthenic exercises in the morning, however, should not cause any physical discomfort.

If the early morning is the only time you have free to exercise, you should get up earlier so that you have an hour or two between breakfast and exercise. If that is not possible, eat a light breakfast of juice and toast before exercising.

Many individuals are not affected by the time of day that they exercise. The time to exercise should depend upon convenience and your psychological motivation. Many people enjoy exercise late in the afternoon, when they are through with work and when they feel more relaxed.

Exercise Precautions

Be familiar with the following exercise precautions before beginning your cardiovascular program:

1. Get a thorough physical examination before starting your conditioning program.
2. If fatigue lasts two hours or more following an exercise session, the program is too rigorous. Reduce your level of exercise.
3. Alcohol and exercise do not mix. Alcohol constricts the coronary vessels of the heart muscle.
4. Cigarette smoking limits oxygen exchange in the lungs, thus preventing a high level of fitness attainment.
5. Remember to use your heart rate as a guide to the intensity of the exercise.
6. Spasmodic exercise may be detrimental to your health. Three to five exercise sessions a week are minimal for optimum benefit.

If any of the following symptoms occur while you are exercising, stop exercising and consult a physician before continuing your exercise program:

1. Fluttering, palpitating, missed, or extra heartbeats, sudden bursts of rapid heartbeats, or a sudden slowing of rapid pulse
2. Pressure or pain in the center of the chest, left arm, fingers, or throat
3. Dizziness, fainting, nausea, cold sweat, or light-headedness

During Exercise

While exercising, you may be fortunate enough to experience the "second-wind phenomenon," or you may have the misfortune of getting a "stitch in your side." During exercise, you must always be aware of how you are feeling and any body signals that may indicate that you are overdoing it.

Second Wind

The **second wind** is a familiar phenomenon to individuals involved in endurance activities, such as long-distance running, cycling, and skiing, and who are in excellent cardiovascular condition. It is generally evidenced by a feeling of relief from the effects of fatigue.

While little research has been conducted in the area of second wind, several factors have been evaluated. There appears to be a psychological mental set that many athletes look forward to that gives them relief from the feelings of discomfort produced by high levels of chemical fatigue products and carbon dioxide in the blood. Other factors that may contribute to the second wind are increased efficiency of circulation, better buffering of the acids produced by muscle contractions, better circulation to the extremities, and a higher metabolic efficiency to the cells. Any of these factors could result in some relief from the symptoms of fatigue.

Stitch in Side

A stitch in the side is pain felt in the lower part of the rib cage or in the upper abdominal area. The pain may be caused by a lack of blood supply to the muscles responsible for the breathing movements. Sometimes, the diaphragm also will experience reduced blood flow during rapid breathing. Or the stitch may be caused by reduced blood supply to the liver during rigorous physical activity. Eating or drinking just prior to rigorous exercise is another possible explanation for stomach or intestinal cramps.

During rigorous physical exercise, the muscles are contracting very rapidly and have a tendency to fatigue. As a result of reduced blood supply, they may go into spasm, which results in pain. Not much can be done to reduce the pain, aside from discontinuing exercise.

No matter what kind of cardiovascular shape you are in, there is always a risk of getting a stitch. Good cardiovascular conditioning, however, does give you some protection because the muscles for breathing, like other muscles in the body, can be conditioned through exercise. The stronger and more efficient your breathing muscles, the more ably they can maintain rapid breathing for longer periods of time during exercise.

Body Signals of Overexercise

When you go beyond the normal limits of physical ability and don't give your body a chance to recover—in other words, when you overexercise—you could fall prey to a number of undesirable symptoms, such as dizziness, severe breathlessness, tightness in the chest or a feeling of weight on the chest, nausea, or a loss of muscular control. If any of these symptoms occur, you should stop exercising immediately.

Common problems *after* a session of overexercising include sleeping difficulties, joint pain, soreness, a feeling of heaviness, loss of appetite, a feeling of anxiety or nervousness, an inability to relax, and reduced skill performance. If these symptoms appear, you should reduce your exercise both in intensity and duration until the symptoms disappear. If any of these symptoms persist, it is important to check with a physician.

After Exercise

After exercise, your body needs both a cooling-down period and then a recovery period before any further exercise is undertaken.

Cooling Down

Cooling down may be defined as the continuation of exercise at a low intensity following a rigorous workout, which allows the body to adjust to a resting state. During rigorous exercise, the muscles utilize over 85 percent of all the blood pumped out of the heart. Even after you stop exercising, the heart continues to provide large amounts of blood until energy has been restored to the muscles. The amount of blood pumped out of the heart is ultimately dependent on the amount of blood returned to the heart by the circulatory system. The blood that is in the lower part of the body below the heart is dependent upon muscle contractions and breathing movements for its return to the heart via the veins. When you stop exercising, blood is still being sent to the muscles. However, if you become sedentary immediately after exercise, the muscle contractions necessary to send blood back to the heart are minimal, thus allowing blood to pool in the lower extremities. This results in a reduced amount of blood returning to the heart and possible interruption to the cardiac cycle, which could lead to dangerous complications. Cooling down also helps to prevent muscle soreness and dizziness and reduces the amounts of biochemical fatigue products in the blood. It is therefore vital to continue slow, relaxed walking after the end of your exercise for approximately five minutes or until your heart rate is below one hundred beats per minute.

Generally, the time required for the heart rate to return to normal after exercise depends upon the intensity of the exercise, the length of the exercise period, and your physical condition. Following very rigorous exercise, the heart rate may remain slightly elevated for as long as two hours. If you are in good physical condition, however, recovery will be rapid. Individuals in poor physical condition will have heart rates that tend to return to normal more slowly after exercise.

Recovery Duration

Your body must have a chance to recover from intensive, rigorous physical exercise. Some individuals may take twelve to fourteen hours to recover from exercise; others may take twenty-four hours or more. Periods of recovery from very prolonged exercise, such as marathon running, long-distance running, and skiing, for fit individuals can be anywhere from ten to forty-eight hours before the amount of muscle glycogen returns to normal. Intermittent exercise, such as interval training (running with rest intervals), where exercise is not continuous, may require anywhere from five to twenty-four hours of recovery before a complete supply of glycogen is restored to the muscles. If you don't allow your body time to recover from exercise, you may counteract any training effects that you are trying to achieve.

The best advice is to give your body plenty of time to recover. Especially in the early stages of your exercise program, twenty-four to forty-eight hours between exercise sessions is preferable. If you find yourself waking up in the morning overly exhausted, it is an indication that you should reduce your exercise intensity level and allow more recovery time.

Increase in Heart Size

Physical training over long periods of time results in a dramatic increase in heart size, along with a number of microscopic cellular changes of unknown significance. This increase in the size of the heart muscle is called **cardiac hypertrophy.** In the past, cardiac hypertrophy has been referred to as "athlete's heart" to differentiate it from a heart enlarged by disease (see chapter 11).

Through training, it is possible for the heart to increase in size as much as 15 percent. This is an obvious advantage to athletes because the stronger contraction from the larger heart muscle results in an increased volume of blood released by the heart. (The cardiac output is how much blood can be pumped out as the result of each stroke from the left ventricle multiplied by the heart rate.) As a result, cardiac hypertrophy is associated with an increased ability to deliver blood to the working muscles.

Recent evidence suggests that cardiac hypertrophy is manifested in different ways, depending on whether you engage in endurance activities or nonendurance activities. Endurance or aerobic activities, such as long-distance running and swimming, produce an increase in the size of the heart's left ventricular cavity, enabling it to hold more blood, and a slight increase in the thickness of the heart's wall. Nonendurance or anaerobic activities, such as weight lifting or sprinting,

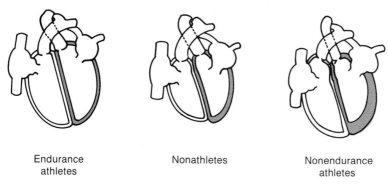

Endurance   Nonathletes   Nonendurance
athletes   athletes

Figure 5.2 Cardiac hypertrophy. From
Sports Physiology, by Edward L. Fox,
copyright © 1979 by Saunders College
Publishing/Holt, Rinehart and Winston.
Reprinted by permission of CBS
College Publishing.

produce a greater increase in the ventricular walls' thickness than produced by aerobic training, with no increase in the size of the ventricular cavity (see figure 5.2). In endurance activities, large volumes of blood must be delivered to the working muscles. If a person has a large left ventricular cavity resulting from training, this ensures sufficient blood to sustain the activity. Anaerobic activities, on the other hand, place great stress on the heart and sudden increases in blood pressure. The increased thickness of the heart muscle as a result of training prepares the heart to deal with these additional stresses and perform more efficiently.

Cardiovascular Training Effects

Individuals who participate in regular cardiovascular physical activities benefit in a number of ways (see table 5.2). In general, only a few weeks after beginning training, your resting heart rate may decrease. In addition, cardiovascular exercise results in an increased supply of red blood cells and hemoglobin, which increases the blood's oxygen-carrying capacity. This enables you to more efficiently supply your working muscles with energy and increases your ability to eliminate metabolic waste products, thus delaying the onset of fatigue.

For physiological changes to occur in the cardiovascular system, the oxygen system and the metabolism of the muscle cells must be appropriately stimulated. For example, young individuals who begin an aerobic exercise program three to five times a week for approximately thirty to sixty minutes a day and who train at about 70 percent of their maximum heart rate (140 to 150 beats per minute) can expect a 20 to 30 percent improvement in the oxygen carried in the blood

Table 5.2 Cardiovascular Training Effects

Cardiovascular training increases	Cardiovascular training produces	Cardiovascular training decreases
Tolerance to stress	Lower resting heart rate	Obesity-adiposity
Arterial oxygen content	Physical conditioning of muscles	Arterial blood pressure
Electron transport activity		Heart rate
Efficiency of the heart	Greater oxygen utilization	Vulnerability to dysrhythmias
Blood vessel size	Greater stroke volume	Stress response
Efficiency of blood circulation	Lower heart rate for submaximal work	Need of heart muscle for oxygen

within approximately two months. If you choose to keep constant the amount of time per workout, you can increase the intensity of the workout to ensure improvements in cardiovascular endurance.

It should be noted, however, that a number of individual genetic and physiological factors contribute to the individual's potential to increase cardiovascular endurance.

Key Terms

Aerobic Exercises Continuous, rigorous exercise lasting beyond one to two minutes, such as jogging, long-distance swimming, cycling, and cross-country skiing; exercises utilizing oxygen

Anaerobic Exercises All-out exercise lasting one to two minutes, such as weight lifting, sprinting, tennis, handball, squash, volleyball, and racquetball; exercises performed in the absence of oxygen

Cardiac Arrhythmia Irregular contractions of the heart muscle

Cardiac Hypertrophy Increase in the size of the heart muscle

Cooling Down Continuation of exercise at a low intensity following a rigorous workout, which allows the body to adjust to a resting state

Duration Amount of time utilized for each exercise bout

Frequency Number of exercise bouts per week

Heart Rate Training Effect The proper intensity level of an endurance training program (approximately 70 percent of maximum heart rate); related to maximum oxygen uptake

Intensity The level of physiological stress on the body during exercise

Maximum Oxygen Uptake The greatest amount of oxygen utilized by the cells during maximum exercise per unit of time

Perceived Exertion An indirect method of determining heart rate

Second Wind General feeling of relief from the effects of fatigue

Stroke Volume Amount of blood pumped out of the left or right ventricle each time it contracts

6

Starting Your Cardiovascular Fitness Program

Getting Started

Now that you have had a chance to evaluate your fitness level and have shifted your motivation into high gear, you are ready to begin an aerobic fitness program. From the programs presented in this chapter, select an aerobic exercise program that is appropriate for your aerobic fitness level (chapter 3) and your computed heart rate training effect level (chapter 5).

If you have been sedentary for a number of months and are just beginning a program, use 60 percent instead of 70 percent as your heart rate training effect level until you have exercised for four to six weeks. Also, expect a little muscle stiffness and soreness the first few days. This is your body's way of telling you that it has been a long time between workouts. The discomfort should go away in a short time. Follow closely the warm-up principles and procedures presented in chapter 4, and don't take any shortcuts. Remember to cool down after exercise no matter how good you feel.

Make minor modifications to the intensity and duration of the aerobic program you select, depending on how well you respond to the exercise. Time is on your side; don't overstress yourself the first few weeks. Check your heart rate periodically throughout the exercise to make sure that you remain at the proper intensity level. If your heart rate goes over the heart rate training effect level, slow your pace or walk a little further between repetitions. If, however, you find yourself below your heart rate training effect level, you may want to quicken your pace. After a few weeks of monitoring your heart rate, you will become an expert at determining the proper intensity required to maintain your training effect level.

If you have difficulty completing the repetitions in any of the recommended programs, go back to the previous level until you successfully achieve the new level without undue stress.

At the end of six to eight weeks, reevaluate your cardiovascular fitness level and replot your fitness paradigm and profile (figures 3.16 and 3.17).

It is important to remember that the target heart rate intensity and the goals listed in this chapter are only guidelines. Continuing to persevere toward a predetermined intensity when your body is telling you that you are overdoing it is not only foolish but dangerous.

Tune into your body's signals while exercising. You know more or less how you feel and how your body is responding to the exercise. You can tell whether or not you have a feeling of well-being. This is especially important when exercising with a group. Don't let group pressure force you to do things that your body says is too much. You are the best judge as to what your body is capable of doing. Establish your own pace and goals.

If you feel sick or overly fatigued, don't continue your exercise until you are feeling better or the cause of your indisposition has been determined. A general principle is: Don't exercise to the point where you feel exhausted, unduly winded, or have pain or discomfort in your chest area. Appropriate individualized exercises should make you feel good, not sick.

No single exercise can universally meet the needs of all individuals. We all have various levels of skill, motivation, and fitness. You must choose the activity that best meets your interests and capabilities. No matter what exercise program you select, however, it should follow the sequence and fall within the time ranges shown in figure 6.1.

Aerobic Exercise Programs

Four aerobic exercise programs are outlined in this chapter: (1) walking/jogging, (2) cycling, (3) rope jumping, and (4) swimming.

Walking/Jogging

Someone once said that the trouble with walking is that it is too easy. Walking is so natural and relaxing that most people don't consider it a form of exercise or understand that it can be beneficial to their health. Walking is appealing because no special equipment is needed, no training is necessary, and you can walk anywhere. Walking uses large muscle groups essential for fitness. It is rhythmic, self-pacing, pleasant, and safe.

Jogging is a slow run in which your heel hits the ground first and then your toes. Avoid running on your toes since this can injure your lower back or joints.

When you first start your walking/jogging exercise program, do not attempt to get yourself in shape in one day. Build up to it gradually. Your intensity and frequency should depend on your individual goals. You might spend two to four weeks walking before you even start to jog. Because this gives your body a chance to gradually accommodate to the exercise load, you probably will have no difficulty when you begin jogging.

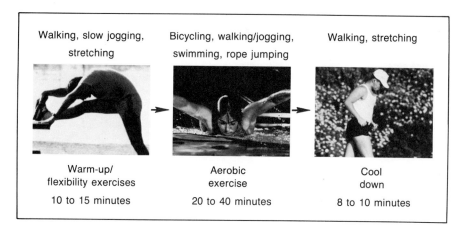

Walking, slow jogging, stretching	Bicycling, walking/jogging, swimming, rope jumping	Walking, stretching
Warm-up/ flexibility exercises	Aerobic exercise	Cool down
10 to 15 minutes	20 to 40 minutes	8 to 10 minutes

Figure 6.1 Sequence and time ranges for basic fitness programs. Photograph by: left and right: Berg & Assoc./Kirk Schlea, middle: Jon Jacobson

Table 6.1 lists recommended walking and jogging regimens that will get you started. For adults whose fitness level falls within the "very poor" to "average" range, the sixteen-week walking/jogging program outlined in table 6.2 is recommended.

Cycling

Long-distance cycling is excellent for building cardiovascular endurance and also for increasing the strength and endurance of muscles in the lower extremities. Because cycling is a nonweight bearing activity, there is less chance of injury to the lower body. Also, those individuals with lower-back and leg problems that prohibit jogging can participate in cycling without fear of further injury.

Safety, however, should be a major consideration when cycling. Accident rates for cyclists have risen sharply in recent years. Be sure to wear a helmet and other protective equipment. Try to avoid busy streets and find a bike path or other safe riding areas.

Five miles of cycling at twice the speed of jogging is equivalent to about two miles of jogging. You should aim for a goal of ninety minutes of cycling at approximately 15 MPH, three to five days a week. Table 6.3 (p. 82) lists recommended levels of cycling according to your fitness category.

Rope Jumping

Rope jumping does an excellent job of stimulating the cardiovascular system. The exercise should be about twenty minutes long for best results.

Table 6.1 Walking/Jogging Program for Cardiovascular Fitness

Fitness category	Starting level
"Very poor" to "poor"	1 to 2
"Average" to "good"	2 to 3
"Very good" to "excellent"	4 to 5
"Superior"	5 to 7

Level	Exercise	Heart rate training effect level (intensity)	Frequency	Duration
1	Walk for 10 to 20 minutes.	60%	3 days	2 to 4 weeks
2	Walk fast for 15 to 20 minutes.	60%	3 days	2 to 4 weeks
3	Jog 100 yards and then walk 300 yards. Repeat four times. Add one repetition for each succeeding exercise session. When you reach eight repetitions, move to level 4. (approximately 30 minutes)	60%	3 days	2 to 3 weeks
4	Jog 200 yards and then walk 200 yards. Repeat four times. Add one repetition for each succeeding exercise session. When you reach eight repetitions, move to level 5. (approximately 28 minutes)	60%	3 to 4 days	2 to 3 weeks
5	Jog 400 yards and then walk 400 yards. Repeat four times. Add one repetition for each succeeding exercise session. When you reach eight repetitions, move to level 6. (approximately 26 minutes)	70%	3 to 4 days	2 to 3 weeks
6	Jog 800 yards and then walk 400 yards. Repeat four times. Add one repetition for every other exercise session. When you reach six repetitions, move to level 7. (approximately 22 minutes)	70%	3 to 5 days	2 to 3 weeks
7	Jog 1,200 yards and then walk 600 yards. Repeat two times. Add one repetition for every other exercise session. When you reach four repetitions, move to level 8. (approximately 22 minutes)	70%	3 to 5 days	2 to 3 weeks
8	Jog 1 mile in 10 minutes and then walk 3 minutes. Then jog 1 mile again in 10 to 12 minutes.	70%	3 to 5 days	2 to 3 weeks
9	Jog 1½ miles in 15 minutes and then walk 6 to 8 minutes. Then jog again 1½ miles in 15 to 18 minutes.	70%	3 to 5 days	2 to 3 weeks
10	Jog 2 miles in 20 minutes.	70%	3 to 5 days	2 to 3 weeks
11	Jog 2 miles in 18 minutes.	70%	3 to 5 days	2 to 3 weeks
12	Jog 2 miles in 16 minutes.	70%	3 to 5 days	2 to 3 weeks
13	Jog 2 miles in 14 minutes.	70%	3 to 5 days	2 to 3 weeks
14	Continue at level 13 to maintain lifetime fitness.			

Table 6.2 Sixteen-Week Walking/Jogging Program for Adults with Low-Level Fitness

Weeks 1 and 2

For the first two weeks, walk at a brisk pace for 10 minutes each day, 3 to 5 days a week. If you become tired after the first 3 to 5 minutes of walking, walk slowly for the remainder of the 10 minutes. (50 percent heart rate training effect level)

Weeks 3 and 4

Walk briskly for 15 minutes. If you feel tired after the first 6 to 8 minutes, walk slowly for 3 to 4 minutes and then walk briskly for the remainder of the 15 minutes. (60 percent heart rate training effect level)

Weeks 5 and 6

Walk briskly for 10 minutes, then walk slowly for 3 to 4 minutes, and then walk briskly again for the final 10 minutes. (60 percent heart rate training effect level)

Week 7

Jog 30 yards and then walk for 2 minutes. Repeat nine times. (60 percent heart rate training effect level)

Week 8

Jog 60 yards and then walk for 2 minutes. Repeat nine times. (60 percent heart rate training effect level)

Week 9

Jog 110 yards and then walk for 2 minutes. Repeat nine times. (60 percent heart rate training effect level)

Week 10

Jog 130 yards and then walk for 2 minutes. Repeat seven times. (60 percent heart rate training effect level)

Week 11

Jog 250 yards and then walk for 1½ minutes. Repeat four times. (60 percent heart rate training effect level)

Week 12

Jog 500 yards and then walk for 1½ minutes. Repeat three times. (70 percent heart rate training effect level)

Week 13

Jog ½ mile and then walk for 300 yards. Repeat two times. (70 percent heart rate training effect level)

Week 14

Jog ¾ mile and then walk for 3 minutes. Repeat one time. (70 percent heart rate training effect level)

Week 15

Jog 1 mile in approximately 10 minutes and then walk for 3 to 5 minutes. Repeat one time. (70 percent heart rate training effect level)

Week 16

Now you are ready for exercise level 9 presented in table 6.1. Within a few weeks, you should be able to jog the 7-minute mile required at level 13. Remember, don't exceed your 70 percent heart rate training effect level. If you find your heart rate going above your training effect level, slow your pace.

Source: Modified from the President's Council on Physical Fitness: Reporting to the President and the Secretary of Health, Education, and Welfare.

Table 6.3 Cycling Program for Cardiovascular Fitness

Fitness category	Starting level
"Very poor" to "poor"	1
"Average" to "good"	1 to 2
"Very good" to "excellent"	3
"Superior"	3

Level	Exercise	Heart rate training effect level (intensity)	Frequency	Duration
1	Ride for 10 to 25 minutes (10 to 12 MPH).	60%	3 days	4 to 6 weeks
2	Ride for 25 to 30 minutes (12 MPH).	60%	3 days	4 to 6 weeks
3	Ride for 30 to 40 minutes (15 MPH).	70%	3 to 5 days	4 to 6 weeks
4	Ride for 40 to 90 minutes (15 MPH).	70%	3 to 5 days	4 to 6 weeks
5	Continue at level 4 to maintain lifetime fitness.			

A problem with rope jumping, however, is that the continuous stress placed upon the knees and the ankles increases the possibility of injury. Such problems as swollen knees, pain in the lower legs, and stress fractures are not uncommon.

One way to avoid some of these problems is to alternate feet while jumping. Jumping with both feet at once places too much stress on the lower legs. Also, wear a good pair of running shoes with a proper heel support and avoid jumping on very hard surfaces.

Table 6.4 presents a rope-jumping regimen.

Swimming

Swimming is one of the best cardiovascular conditioning exercises. Because swimming is performed in a horizontal position, your body weight is supported by the water, which helps to prevent hip, leg, and back injuries that commonly are associated with running. In addition, swimming is especially appropriate for those who are overweight or handicapped or who have orthopedic problems.

Table 6.4 Rope Jumping (or Bouncing in Place on a Minitrampoline) Program for Cardiovascular Fitness

Fitness category	Starting level
"Very poor" to "poor"	1
"Average" to "good"	2
"Very good" to "excellent"	3
"Superior"	4

Level	Exercise	Heart rate training effect level (intensity)	Frequency	Duration
1	Jump for 30 seconds and then rest for 20 to 40 seconds. Repeat six to eight times. (2 to 5 minutes)	50%	3 days	2 to 4 weeks
2	Jump for 60 seconds and then rest for 60 seconds. Repeat six to eight times. (4 to 10 minutes)	60%	3 days	2 to 4 weeks
3	Jump for 90 seconds and then rest for 15 seconds. Repeat six to eight times. (6 to 12 minutes)	60%	3 days	2 to 4 weeks
4	Jump for 2 minutes and then rest for 30 seconds. Repeat four to eight times. (10 to 25 minutes)	70%	3 to 5 days	2 to 4 weeks
5	Jump for 4 minutes and then rest for 30 seconds. Repeat four to eight times. (15 to 30 minutes)	70%	3 to 5 days	2 to 4 weeks
6	Jump for 8 minutes and then rest for 30 seconds. Repeat one to two times. (15 to 30 minutes)	70%	3 to 5 days	2 to 4 weeks
7	Jump for 10 minutes and then rest for 2 to 3 minutes. Repeat one to two times. (30 minutes)	70%	3 to 5 days	2 to 4 weeks
8	Jump for 10 minutes and then rest for 2 minutes. Repeat two times. (30 minutes)	70%	3 to 5 days	2 to 4 weeks
9	Continue at level 8 to maintain lifetime fitness.			

Because the entire musculature is involved in swimming, energy expenditure is much greater than walking or jogging the same distance. For example, swimming for thirty minutes may produce cardiovascular training effects that would require two to three hours of continuous tennis or badminton.

Table 6.5 outlines a swimming program for cardiovascular fitness.

Table 6.5 Swimming Program for Cardiovascular Fitness

Fitness category	Starting level
"Very poor" to "poor"	1
"Average" to "good"	1 to 2
"Very good" to "excellent"	2 to 3
"Superior"	3 to 4

Level	Exercise	Heart rate training effect level (intensity)	Frequency	Duration
1	Swim 25 yards. Repeat four times with a 30- to 60-second rest between each repetition. While resting at the end of the pool between laps, move your legs slowly as in a walking movement. Add one to two repetitions for each succeeding exercise session until you can do twelve repetitions. Then move on to level 2.	60%	3 days	2 to 4 weeks
2	Swim 50 yards. Repeat four times with a 30- to 60-second rest between each repetition. While resting at the end of the pool between laps, move your legs slowly as in a walking movement. Add one to two repetitions for each succeeding exercise session until you can do twelve repetitions. Then move on to level 3.	60%	3 days	2 to 4 weeks
3	Swim 100 yards. Repeat four times with a 90-second rest between each repetition. While resting at the end of the pool between laps, move your legs slowly as in a walking movement. Add one to two repetitions for each succeeding exercise session until you can do eight repetitions. Then move on to level 4.	60%	3 days	2 to 4 weeks
4	Swim 150 yards. Repeat three times with a 90-second rest between each repetition. While resting at the end of the pool between laps, move your legs slowly as in a walking movement. Add one to two repetitions for each succeeding exercise session until you can do six repetitions. Then move on to level 5.	70%	3 to 5 days	2 to 4 weeks
5	Swim 200 yards. Rest for 60 seconds and then repeat five times.	70%	3 to 5 days	2 to 3 weeks
6	Swim slowly 400 yards. Rest for 2 minutes and then repeat two times.	70%	3 to 5 days	2 to 3 weeks
7	Swim moderately 600 yards.	70%	3 to 5 days	2 to 3 weeks
8	Swim moderately 800 to 1,400 yards.	70%	3 to 5 days	2 to 3 weeks
9	Continue at level 8 to maintain lifetime fitness.			

The major obvious drawback to swimming is that a moderate level of swimming skills is required. However, even those individuals who are not skilled swimmers or who have disabilities that prevent them from leg-supported locomotive movements can improve their cardiovascular fitness by performing the water exercises that follow. The intensity, frequency, and duration of the following exercises should approximate those levels in table 6.5 that are consistent with your fitness category:

1. **Bobbing** Stand in shallow water. Inhale and then duck underwater to a squat position. Blow your air out gradually. Then push off the bottom of the pool to a standing position and inhale.

2. **Treading** Stand in water that is shoulder deep. Bicycle with your feet and scull with your hands palms down to tread water.

3. **Flutter Kicking** Hold onto the side of the pool while lying on your stomach in the water. Kick your legs using a **flutter kick,** a swimming kick executed with the legs horizontal and the knees straight. The legs are alternately moved up and down in rapid succession. Extend your elbows as far as possible.

4. **Climbing** Stand in the water and hold onto the side of the pool with both hands. Place your feet against the side of the pool and walk up and down the pool side.

5. **Knee Flexion** Hold onto the pool side while lying on your back in the water. Bring your knees up to your chest. Hold for five seconds and then extend your knees.

6. **Running in Place** Stand in water that is chest deep and run in place. Maintain your balance by placing your hands palms down in the water, with your elbows flexed ninety degrees.

Other Exercise Options

The four aerobic exercise programs outlined in this chapter—walking/jogging, cycling, rope jumping, and swimming—are excellent for developing cardiovascular fitness. Other exercise options, however, such as jogging in place, dancing, riding a stationary bike, cross-country skiing, and orienteering, can be equally beneficial to the cardiovascular system.

Indoor Exercise Options

A number of beneficial exercises can be performed in your home. Jogging in place for around twenty minutes is excellent exercise. If you find it boring, turn on the television set and watch your favorite program or play some music.

If you don't like running in place, purchase a stationary bicycle. Exercising on a stationary bicycle for twenty-five to thirty minutes a day is an excellent method for training the cardiovascular system. The pedaling rate for training should average between 10 and 14 MPH; however, your best indication of intensity level is your own heart rate response. The stationary bike should be equipped with an odometer and a mechanism for increasing or decreasing resistance to the pedals.

Calisthenics (various gymnastic exercises utilizing both aerobic and anaerobic fitness) or dancing to music are other options. Choreograph your own movements to music and exercise continuously for at least thirty minutes. Check out an aerobic dance class for some tips on movement and music, if it is convenient. Minitrampolines, rowing machines, and even stair climbing also are effective for maintaining continuous and rhythmic exercise. Low impact aerobics (floor exercises to music) may be another option if you have knee or ankle problems.

Cross-Country Skiing

Cross-country skiing is the most demanding cardiovascular exercise in terms of intensity. In addition to the lower body muscles used in running, cross-country skiing requires upper trunk and arm muscles, which add intensity to the cardiovascular system. Therefore, before attempting to participate in this activity, you should have already attained a very high level of cardiovascular endurance. Needless to say, proper equipment and instruction also are essential.

Orienteering

Orienteering is a combination of cross-country running and land navigation. Competitors use only a map and compass to navigate their way between checkpoints along an unfamiliar course. In some European countries, thousands compete in one race. The main objective is the satisfaction of finishing in the allotted time and enjoying and responding to the challenge.

Aesthetic Awareness

An often overlooked factor in exercise, but nevertheless an important one, is the potential for the development of aesthetic awareness. Fortunately, a number of physical activities not only lead to increased fitness but also allow for creative expression. For example, you can create your own expressive floor exercises, explore different kinds of movements in modern jazz and aerobic dance, and choose your own music. Even though there seem to be fewer ways to catch a pass or hit a tennis ball than there are ways to dance or move to music, the opportunity for creativity exists in all sports. The point here is that exercise and staying in shape can develop aspects other than just your cardiovascular fitness.

Tracking Your Cardiovascular Fitness

Aerobic exercise record sheets are provided for you in Appendix B at the back of the book (record sheets B-1 and B-3). Keeping a careful record of your exercise will show you the steady advances you make toward cardiovascular fitness.

Key Terms

Calisthenics   Various gymnastic exercises utilizing both aerobic and anaerobic fitness

Flutter Kick   A swimming kick executed with the legs horizontal and the knees straight—the legs are alternately moved up and down in rapid succession

Orienteering   A combination of cross-country running and land navigation

Muscle Strength and Endurance

Importance of Muscle Strength and Endurance

The terms *muscle strength* and *muscle endurance* are often confused, and it is important to differentiate between them. **Muscle strength** is the amount of force that can be exerted by a muscle group for one movement or repetition. **Muscle endurance** is the ability of the muscle group to maintain a continuous contraction or repetition over a period of time. The muscle system is at the foundation of all physical exercise. No matter what activity you participate in, your muscle strength and endurance determine your exercise limits.

Body motion, the beating of the heart, breathing movements, movements of the bones, balance, and posture are all brought about by the contraction of muscles. Yet, muscles are not independent from the rest of the body systems, and conditioning is not limited solely to the muscles. Your muscles' ability to do work is totally dependent upon the efficiency of the heart, blood vessels, and lungs in providing energy and waste product elimination. Muscles, the heart, blood vessels, and the lungs are simultaneously conditioned because of their interdependence.

Your main goal in conditioning the muscle system is not to build big, bulky muscles like the bodybuilders seen on television or the weight lifters in the Olympics. These individuals have trained rigorously for years in highly specialized weight programs to develop their special qualities. Your primary goal is to increase the strength and endurance of your muscles so that they become more efficient in dealing with the everyday demands placed upon them. Whether it's mowing the grass in the backyard, moving the filing cabinet at the office, or meeting the unforeseen physical demands of an emergency situation, well-conditioned muscles enable you to make the necessary adaptations more effectively and without injury.

Research on muscles has advanced rapidly in the past ten years in such areas as muscle fatigue, fiber type, weight-resistance training, and injury. Even with these advances, some confusion still exists with regard to the most efficient techniques for increasing strength and endurance. However, research indicates that certain training procedures produce greater muscle efficiency than others.

Before discussing the three basic weight-resistance programs, we examine the basic principles of weight-resistance training and how to determine the amount of resistance to use for training.

Basic Principles of Weight-Resistance Training

Four basic principles of weight-resistance training should be followed to derive the maximum strength and endurance gains from the training regimen: (1) overload, (2) progressive resistance, (3) specificity, and (4) allowing for adequate recovery.

Overload

Muscle strength only develops when muscles are **overloaded**—forced to contract at maximum or near maximum tension. Muscle contractions at these tension levels produce physiological changes in the muscles, resulting in strength gains. If muscles are not overloaded to this degree, they do not increase in strength or in size (hypertrophy). Muscles adapt only to the load they are subjected to. A maximum overload results in maximum strength gains, whereas a minimum overload produces only minimum strength gains.

Progressive Resistance

As muscle strength increases from training, the initial training load no longer provides adequate strength gains. If the intensity of the training load is not increased, only existing strength levels are maintained. Therefore, the intensity of the load must be progressively increased to ensure future strength gains, a concept known as **progressive resistance.**

Specificity

The demands of the exercise must be sufficient to force muscles to adapt, and the subsequent muscle adaptations are specific to the type of training performed, a concept known as **specificity.** For example, aerobic activity develops aerobic capacity, and anaerobic activity develops anaerobic capacity.

Recent research indicates that muscle adaptations are specific to the type of training performed because exercise not only affects muscles but also nerve control of muscles. The nerve pathways appear to become more efficient with continued exercise. The efficiency, however, is specific only to the particular exercise.

Research also indicates that the joint angle of exercise, the type of exercise (that is, isotonic, isometric, or isokinetic), and the speed and range of movement all produce a variety of specific muscle adaptations.

Allowing for Adequate Recovery

Progressive training becomes less effective when muscles become fatigued since the training stimulus cannot be maintained at maximum level. Also, overloading a fatigued muscle may lead to soreness and injury. Therefore, follow three simple rules:

1. Exercise large muscle groups before smaller ones. Movements become fatiguing when the small muscles involved in the movement are fatigued. For example, before performing standing overhead lifts with free weights, first exercise the leg muscles and then the lower arm muscles.
2. Arrange your strength exercises so that successive exercises only minimally affect the muscle groups that were just trained previously.
3. Allow forty-eight hours between strength exercises for complete physiological recovery.

Determining the Amount of Resistance

Muscle strength is most effectively developed when muscles are overloaded—that is, exercised against maximum or near maximum resistance. Heavy resistance forces muscles to contract maximally, thus stimulating the physiological adaptations that lead to increased strength.

Generally, to increase muscle strength, the intensity should be near maximum with a low number of repetitions, and to gain muscle endurance, the intensity should be lower with a high number of repetitions. The intensity level for strength gains is believed to be between one and six repetitions maximum; for endurance gains, it is believed to be over six repetitions maximum. One repetition maximum (RM) is the maximum load that you can lift successfully *once* through the full range of movement, two repetitions maximum (2 RM) is the amount you can lift successfully *twice* through the full range of movement, and so on.

When beginning a weight-training program, it is best to select an intensity around 10 to 12 RM. This reduces your chance of injury and gives you time to acquire the proper form required for lifting. After several weeks, you may work up to an intensity of 1 to 6 RM. As training progresses, you will experience strength gains, and as a result, your original repetition maximum will have to be increased. Therefore, you should determine a new repetition maximum approximately every two weeks. Keep in mind, however, that individuals vary widely in their response to strength programs, and exceptions to these training principles are not uncommon.

Table 7.1 Recommendations for Increasing Strength and Endurance through Isotonic Exercise

Frequency	Three to five days per week		
Duration	Six weeks minimum		
Intensity	Beginners: Strength: Endurance:	10–12 RM load 1–6 RM load 12–14 RM load	
Repetitions*	Beginners: Strength: Endurance:	4–8 repetitions 3–6 repetitions 12–14 repetitions	(Three sets each exercise) (Three sets each exercise) (Three sets each exercise)

*A repetition is the number of continuous contractions per set or group.

Weight-Resistance Programs

Weight-resistance programs can involve isotonic exercise, isometric exercise, and isokinetic exercise.

Isotonic Exercise

Isotonic exercise is exercise that is performed against resistance while the load remains constant, with the resistance varying with the angle of the joint (for example, lifting free weights (barbells) or weight stacks, such as used on the universal gym). The free weights seem to be the most popular among today's athletes, who are convinced that the way to higher levels of athletic performance is through increases in strength, power, and endurance.

If you are a beginner starting your first isotonic weight program, table 7.1 recommends that you start at an intensity load of 10 to 12 RM. To determine your 10 to 12 RM, you must find a weight that you can lift successfully twelve times (using the higher RM) through the full range of movement before you fatigue. For example, using a biceps curl (figure 7.1), you might find after a little trial and error that you are able to curl thirty pounds twelve consecutive times before fatiguing. Therefore, thirty pounds would be your 12 RM for this exercise. According to table 7.1, you should complete three sets of four to eight repetitions for each set with the thirty-pound (12 RM) load. Remember, you must determine your repetition maximum (intensity) for each specific isotonic exercise. Table 7.1 recommends specific intensity and repetition levels for increasing strength and endurance through isotonic exercise.

Variations of isotonic exercise include speed loading, eccentric loading, and plyometric loading.

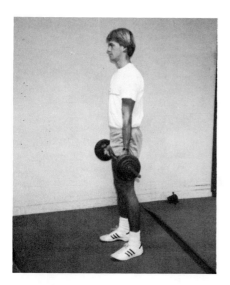 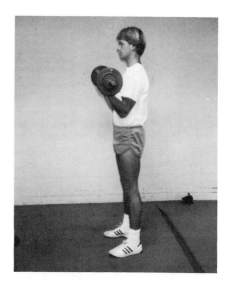

Figure 7.1 Biceps curl (upper, lower arm). Grasp the bar with your hands shoulder-width apart, using an underhand grip. Bring the bar to a position of rest against your thigh, with your elbow fully extended and your feet spread shoulder-width apart. Using only your arms, raise the bar to your chest and then return to the starting position. Keep your back straight and always return to a position where your elbows are fully extended.

Speed Loading

Speed loading occurs when the resistance is moved as rapidly as possible. This technique is believed to be inferior to the more commonly practiced constant resistant isotonic exercise for gaining strength since not enough tension is produced for a training effect. However, many athletes use this technique during competition when maximum power is desired.

Eccentric Loading

Eccentric loading is sometimes referred to as a negative contraction because the muscle lengthens as it develops tension. Examples would be letting yourself down slowly from a chin-up or extending your elbow slowly from a flexed position while holding a weight in your hand. This type of exercise tends to produce more muscle soreness than other techniques. It is not superior to other isotonic methods and is used mainly as an addition to other training techniques.

Plyometric Loading

Plyometric loading requires that the muscles be loaded suddenly and then forced to stretch before the contraction for movement occurs. This type of exercise has gained some popularity among volleyball players, skiers, discus throwers, and

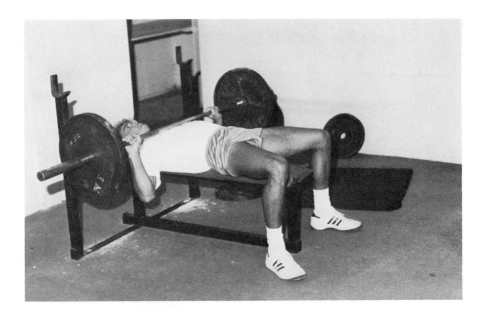

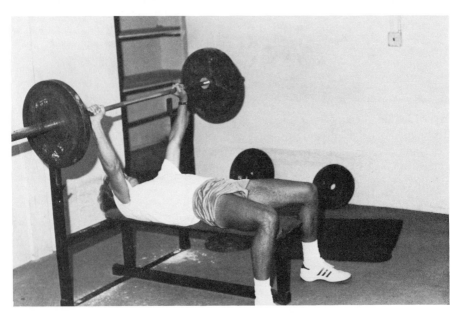

Figure 7.2 Bench press (chest). From a supine position on a bench, take the weight with an overhand grip, hands shoulder-width apart, elbows fully extended. Lower the weight to your chest and then return to your starting position.

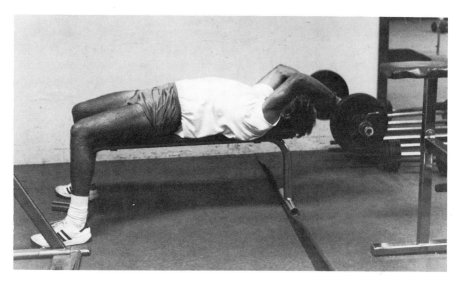

Figure 7.3 Bent-arm pullover (chest). Lying supine on a bench, with the barbell overhead in an overhand grasp, hands shoulder-width apart, lower the barbell slowly over and behind the head as far back as possible and then return to the starting position.

shot-putters. An example would be to jump from a bench to the floor and then immediately back onto the bench. This exercise has been shown to increase strength and jumping ability. However, anyone who attempts this exercise should be aware of the possibility of injury to the ankles and knee joints.

Prescribed Strength Exercises Using Free Weights

Figures 7.1–7.9 illustrate isotonic exercises for increasing strength with the use of free weights. If you do not have access to free weights, the exercises illustrated in figures 7.10–7.13 can be very useful in increasing strength.

Universal Exercise Stations

Figures 7.14–7.20 illustrate isotonic exercises that can be used on universal exercise stations.

Isometric Exercise

An **isometric exercise** is a contraction performed against a fixed or immovable resistance, where tension is developed in the muscle but there is no change in the length of the muscle or the angle of the joint. This also is referred to as a static contraction. An example would be holding a heavy weight in one position for a fixed amount of time.

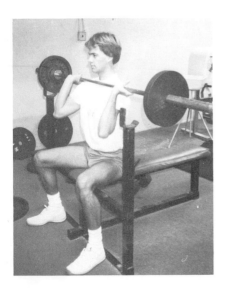

Figure 7.4 Shoulder press (shoulders, upper arms). Sit with your feet shoulder-width apart on the floor. Then bend your knees to forty-five degrees and grasp the bar with an overhand grip, hands spread shoulder-width apart. With your elbows under the bar, lift the weight over your head and return to your starting position.

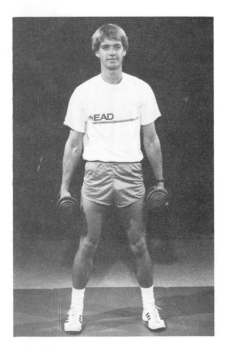

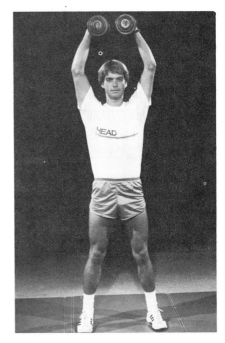

Figure 7.5 Lateral arm raise (shoulder). With one dumbbell in each hand, arms hanging down to your sides, raise both of your arms out to the side of your body and then to an overhead position, keeping your elbows locked in extension. Then return to your starting position.

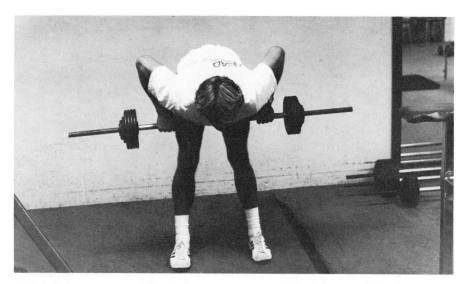

Figure 7.6 Bent-over rowing (shoulder, girdle). Flex your knees at a forty-five-degree angle and bend over from your hips until your back is parallel to the floor. With your arms extended, grab the barbell with your hands pronated. Lift the barbell to your chest and then return.

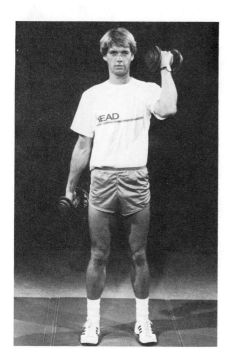

Figure 7.7 Zottman curl (upper arm, forearm). With a weight in each hand, curl your hands alternately, palms up, above the shoulder, and then extend to the rear. When extending to the rear, rotate your forearm so that the palm faces the front.

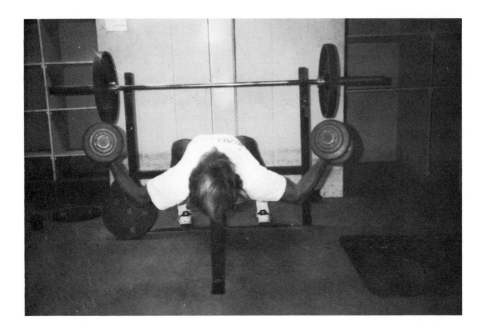

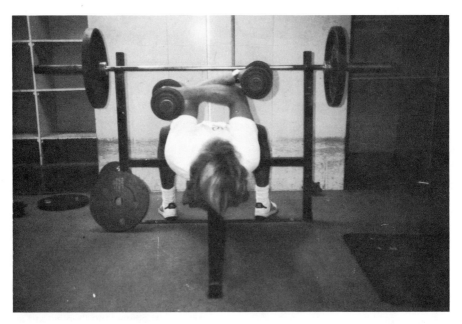

Figure 7.8 Bent-arm lateral (chest and arms). With your elbows bent and your hands palms up, bring the weights from a lateral position and cross them in front of your body.

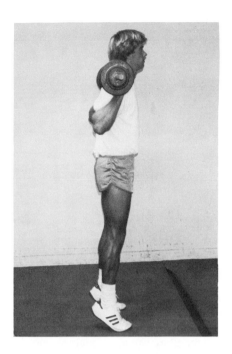

Figure 7.9 Heel raise (calf muscles). Rest the barbell on your shoulders, with the palms of your hands facing forward. Shift your body weight to the balls of your feet and then raise your heels off the floor.

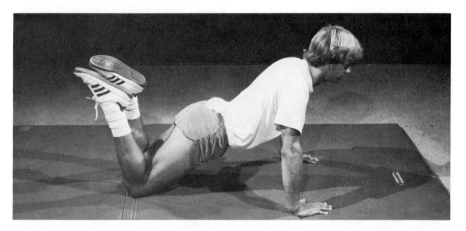

Figure 7.10 Modified push-up. If you have limited upper-body strength, start with the modified push-up. Lie flat on your stomach with your hands in a position to push the trunk upward and with your legs bent upward at the knees. Keeping your back straight and in line with your buttocks, raise your trunk until your arms are fully extended at the elbows. Lower your body to a position where your chest just touches the floor and then push back up to the fully extended position. This exercise is to be done with the arms only, so immobilize the rest of your body. Start with ten repetitions.

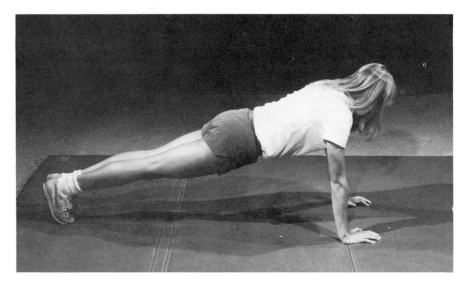

Figure 7.11 Full push-up. Once you have mastered thirty repetitions of the modified push-up, you have the strength to perform the full push-up. Perform this exercise exactly as you did the modified version, except now use your toes—not your knees—as the point of support. This forces you to lift a greater percentage of your body weight. Start with ten repetitions and increase to thirty.

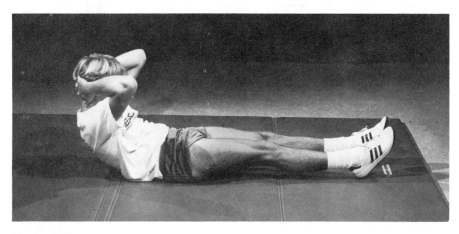

Figure 7.12 Head-and-shoulder curl. Lie on your back with your legs fully extended in front. Place your hands behind either your head or your neck. Slowly curl the head and shoulders up to about a forty-five-degree angle. Hold this position for five seconds and then return to the starting position. Start with ten repetitions and increase to thirty.

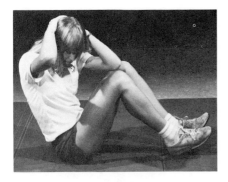

Figure 7.13 Bent-knee sit-up. Lie on your back with your knees bent to a ninety-degree angle, feet flat on the floor. With your hands behind your head, curl your head, shoulders, and trunk slowly upward to a full sitting position and touch one of your knees with the opposite elbow. Return slowly to the starting position and repeat. Start with ten repetitions and gradually build up to forty.

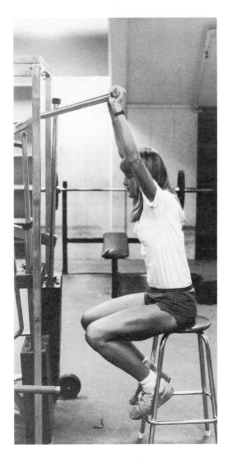

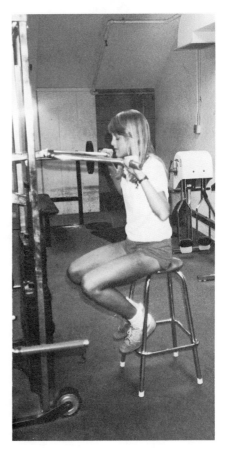

Figure 7.14 Pull down. Start in a kneeling or sitting position. With your hands palms down, pull the bar down to your chest and then slowly return it to the starting position.

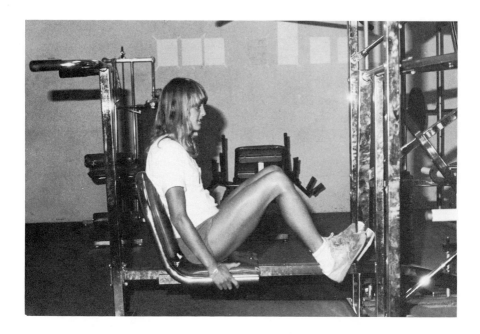

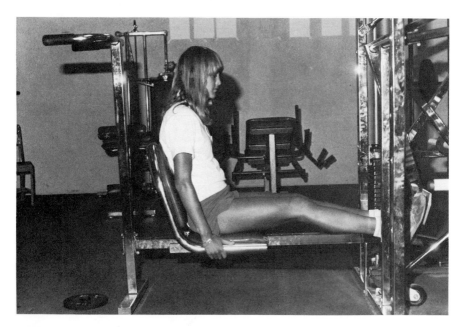

Figure 7.15 Leg press. Push the leg
pedal away from you by extending your
knees.

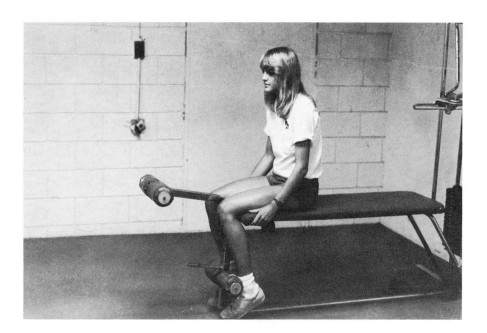

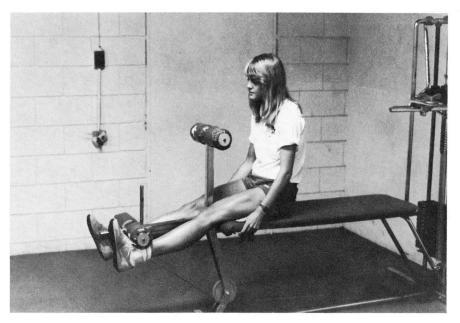

Figure 7.16 Knee extension. Grasp the bench with both of your hands while in a sitting position. Hook the top of your ankles behind the lower bars. Pull the lever up by straightening your knees.

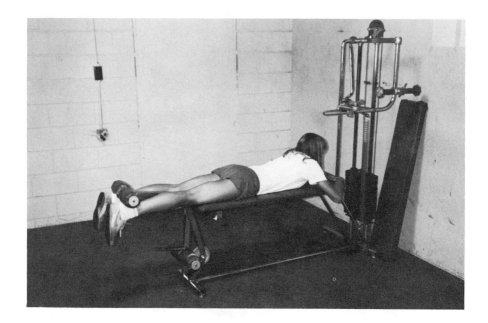

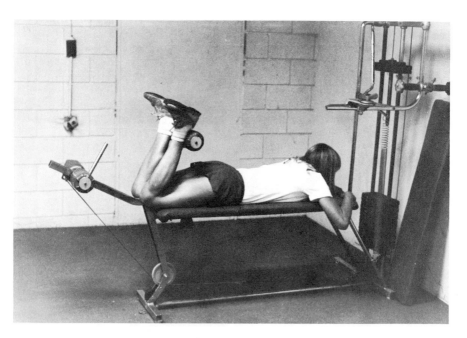

Figure 7.17 Knee flexion. Lie on your abdomen on the leg machine bench. Hook the back of your ankles behind the upper bar. Pull the lever up by bending your knees as far as possible.

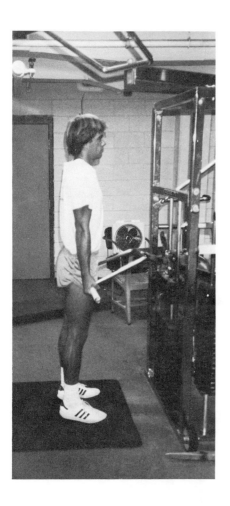

Figure 7.18 Elbow flexion curl. Grasp the bar using an underhand grip with your hands shoulder-width apart. Keep your back straight and use only your arms. Raise the bar to your chest and then return to the starting position.

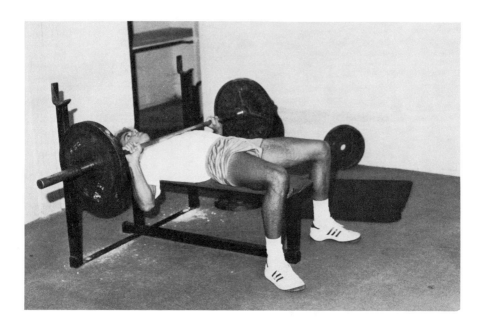

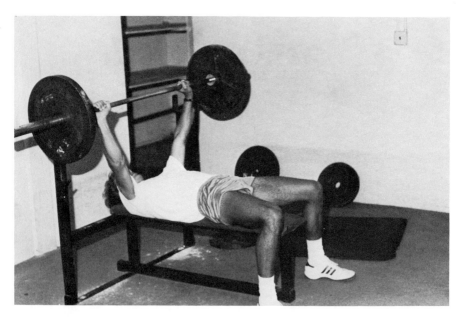

Figure 7.19 Elbow extension (bench press). From a supine position on a bench, take the weight with an overhand grip, hands shoulder-width apart, elbows fully extended. Lower the weight to your chest and then return to your starting position.

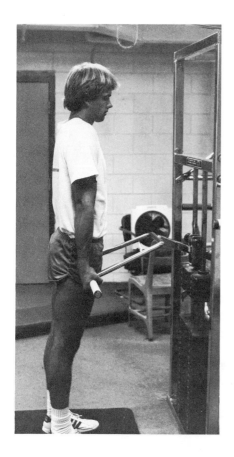

Figure 7.20 Shoulder elevation. Stand with your head and back straight. Grip the bar and lift it with straight arms. Contract your thighs and rotate the points of your shoulder forward and up, then back in a circular fashion.

It appears that with isometric exercise strength development is specific only to the joint angle stimulated during training. As a result, isometric exercise does not increase strength throughout the range of movement. Isometric exercise also may inhibit the ability of the muscle to exert force rapidly, such as is necessary in the shot-put and discus events. In addition, isometric exercise increases pressure in the chest cavity, which results in reduced blood flow to the heart, lungs, and brain, along with increased blood pressure. Consequently, isometric exercises are not recommended for individuals with cardiovascular problems.

Isometric exercise can be utilized by those individuals unable to find free weights or other equipment. It also can be used in conjunction with other weight programs. But unless there are specific reasons for you to limit joint movement or engage in isometric exercise, isotonic exercise is preferred.

Table 7.2 shows the recommended frequency, duration, intensity, and repetitions for increasing strength through isometric exercise. Allow two to three minutes recovery between repetitions if the same muscle group is involved.

Table 7.2 Recommendations for Increasing Strength through Isometric Exercise

Frequency	Three to five days a week
Duration	Six weeks minimum
Intensity	Maximum force held for five to seven seconds
Repetitions	Five to ten

Isokinetic Exercise

An **isokinetic exercise** is a contraction in which the muscle contracts maximally at a constant speed over a full range of the joint movement against a variable resistance. Isokinetic means equal motion, which is interpreted to mean equal rate of motion or equal speed. An isokinetic contraction can only be accomplished with the use of special equipment, such as a minigym that utilizes "accommodating resistance." In other words, the harder you pull, the harder the gym resists you—the resistance is always related to the applied force.

Isokinetic exercise has become popular because it provides a speed-specific indication of the absolute strength of the muscle group being trained, thus enabling one to more closely replicate specific athletic skills. The most effective strength gains have come from slower training speeds of approximately sixty degrees (measure of distance) at one second or less. Recent research, however, has indicated that training at fast speeds of movement generally increases strength at all speeds of movement. Also, isokinetic training at fast speeds of movement increases muscular endurance for movements that require fast speed. Further, isokinetic exercise produces a little less soreness and is considered safer than isometric and isotonic exercise. The refined dials and gauges on isokinetic equipment make it easier to keep track of your load levels and strength gains. Further research still is needed, however, to develop more precise regimens for isokinetic exercise.

Table 7.3 shows the recommended frequency, duration, intensity, repetitions, and speed for increasing strength through isokinetic exercise.

Advantages and Disadvantages of Weight-Resistance Programs

Isotonic, isometric, and isokinetic exercise all have their advantages and disadvantages. As long as the muscle is overloaded, however, it will gain in strength.

Table 7.3 Recommendations for Increasing Strength through Isokinetic Exercise

Frequency	Three to four days per week
Duration	Six weeks
Intensity	Maximum
Repetitions	Eight to fifteen (three sets for each muscle group)
Speed	60 to 300 degrees at one second. The exercise should be similar to the skill being trained for. The training speed should be as fast or faster than the speed involved in the actual athletic event.

Isotonic Exercise

Advantages

1. Generally produces strength gains throughout the full range of movement.
2. Progress in strength gains is easy to evaluate because of numbered free weights and universal stacks.
3. Strength exercises can be developed to duplicate a variety of sports skills.

Disadvantages

1. The equipment is cumbersome.
2. Produces more muscle soreness and greater risk of injury.
3. Most strength gains occur at the weakest point of the movement and are not uniform throughout.

Isometric Exercise

Advantages

1. Little time is required for training.
2. Expensive and cumbersome equipment is not needed.
3. Exercise can be performed anywhere—in home or office or while on vacation.

Disadvantages

1. Strength gains are not produced throughout the full range of movement.
2. Strength gains are difficult to evaluate; that is, no numbered weights or gauges generally are used.
3. Increases the pressure in the chest cavity, causing reduced blood flow to the heart, lungs, and brain.

4. Not as efficient in producing strength gains as isotonic and isokinetic methods.

5. Not effective in producing increases in skilled movements.

6. Motivation is difficult to maintain.

Isokinetic Exercise

Advantages

1. Produces maximum resistance at all ranges of movement.

2. Increases strength throughout the full range of movement.

3. Results in less injury and soreness than isometric and isotonic exercise.

4. The uniqueness of the equipment increases motivation.

5. Strength gains are easy to determine.

Disadvantages

1. The equipment is very expensive, with limited availability.

2. Research is still incomplete with regard to motor patterns and force-velocity relationships.

Other Options for Advanced Strength Training

For advanced strength training, you might want to consider using the Groves super overload method, the rest/pause method, the wipeout method, or the burnout method.

Groves Super Overload Method

To use the Groves super overload method, you first determine your 1 RM for the muscle group to be trained and then add 25 percent more weight. Begin each repetition in the "up" position (for example, the leg press should begin with the legs extended). Relax your muscles so that the joint is bent approximately two or three inches on the first repetition. Continue bringing the weight down until the seventh repetition or until you are unable to return the weight to the "up" position. Complete three sets of seven repetitions every other day. Determine a new 1 RM each week and repeat the procedure.

The Groves super overload method produces large strength gains, especially with bench and leg presses. It is necessary, however, to train a spotter to help you get the weight into the "up" position and back to the "rest" position after the last repetition.

Rest/Pause Method

With the rest/pause method, you first determine your 1 RM for the muscle group to be trained. Perform a single repetition and then rest one to two minutes. Complete a second repetition and then rest again. Continue in this fashion until the muscle group is fatigued.

Wipeout Method

The wipeout method requires that you determine your 1 RM for the muscle group to be trained and then halve that amount. Using ½ RM, complete as many consecutive repetitions as possible until fatigued. Train with a partner in case of premature fatigue.

Burnout Method

With the burnout method, you determine your 1 RM for the muscle group to be trained and then take three-fourths of that amount. Using ¾ RM, complete as many consecutive repetitions as possible until fatigued. Then immediately remove ten pounds and complete as many repetitions as possible until fatigued. Again remove another ten pounds and complete as many repetitions as possible until completely fatigued. Allow no rest periods between repetitions. Train with a partner in case of premature fatigue.

Guidelines for Strength Training

No matter what strength-training program you select, follow these important guidelines:

1. Warm-up should precede all resistance exercise.
2. Muscles must be overloaded—that is, exercised against near maximum resistance—to increase strength and endurance.
3. The overload must be progressive throughout the duration of the program.
4. Larger muscle groups should be exercised before smaller ones.
5. No two successive lifts or exercises should involve the same muscle group.
6. Avoid holding your breath while lifting.
7. Make your exercise interesting. One of the major difficulties of fitness programs—particularly strength programs—is maintaining a high level of motivation. Poorly designed programs lead to boredom and high dropout rates. Be creative in setting up your sequence of exercises; that is, set individual goals, rotate types of strength exercises, and vary the progression of the various exercises.

Weight Lifting Complications and Potential Injuries

When one is involved in lifting maximum weight, there is a possibility of injury. Common problems are hernia (rupture) and injuries to the lower back and joints. In addition, injuries to the bones, muscles, and other tissues are possible. Also, a maximum lift requires a great deal of strength and effort, and sometimes this can put a terrific load upon the heart, requiring it to beat very rapidly. This, however, is a common response and should not be cause for worry.

Three major weight lifting problem areas are the spinal column, the Valsalva maneuver, and muscle soreness.

Spinal Column

The human spinal column is not well-suited for bearing heavy loads unless the back is kept in a very straight position and a normal curvature is maintained. Some movements, such as a two-hands clean military press, where the barbell is lifted over the head, can increase the curvature of the spine and put extreme pressure on the vertebrae and the spinal discs. This type of movement is condemned by many physicians and is considered dangerous in both long- and short-term exercise programs. It is especially dangerous for individuals who are still growing.

Before beginning a weight-resistance program, you should be well aware of the mechanical principles and precautions involved in lifting weight. Or you should at least lift under supervision to safeguard against possible injury.

Valsalva Maneuver

The epiglottis is a piece of cartilage that closes over the top of the windpipe when we swallow so that food does not pass into the windpipe. During weight-resistance training, an individual often exhales against a closed epiglottis, a process called the **Valsalva maneuver.** This type of strain increases pressure within the chest cavity. Because this pressure is placed against the heart and the large veins, it impedes blood flow into the heart (resulting in lowered blood pressure) and increases pressure in the veins going to the extremities and to the head. To counteract the reduced blood flow, the heart rate increases. As soon as the individual relieves the pressure by breathing out, the accumulated blood in the veins rushes into the right ventricle, causing the heart to increase its output and increasing arterial pressure. When this pressure jumps up, the heart rate briefly declines until the resting conditions are reestablished.

For a young person, these sudden increases in pressure and decreases in blood flow to the heart are not dangerous. However, for a person who suffers from heart disease, they could have serious consequences. Individuals involved in weight-resistance training that requires continuous heavy lifting can modify this response by normal breathing while lifting, especially by exhaling during the main contraction.

Muscle Soreness

Muscle soreness after exercise is a very common phenomenon. There are basically two kinds of muscle soreness. One type occurs immediately after exercise and is due partially to the reduced blood supply to the muscles and in some cases to a loss of minerals and increased lactic acid levels. This soreness goes away after a short while.

The other kind of muscle soreness, which has been the subject of considerable research, occurs approximately twenty-four to forty-eight hours after exercise. You no doubt have had that unpleasant experience of waking up in the morning barely able to move after a previous day of exercise. This is usually the result of engaging in either a new exercise or one that you have not participated in for a long time. The exact cause of this kind of muscle soreness is not known.

One theory is that there are minute tears in the muscle that may be caused by eccentric contractions. During this type of contraction, connective tissue associated with the muscle and tendon is stretched. Overextending the muscle can result in damage to the connective tissue of the muscle and to the ends of the muscle (tendons), producing soreness. It is believed that there is less soreness in concentric (shortening) and isometric contractions because only the connective tissue associated with tendons is stretched.

Another theory of muscle soreness is referred to as the spasm theory. When a muscle contracts forcefully during bouncing and ballistic types of movement, the resulting local muscle spasm reduces the blood supply to the muscle (ischemia). Ischemia produces muscle pain, pain produces more spasm, and the cycle continues. A good way to break this cycle and reduce soreness is through stretching exercises. The stretching decreases the spasm and allows blood to flow through the muscle.

Generally, muscle soreness after exercise can be avoided if there is good pre- and post-warm-up exercise, such as stretching. Stretching also can bring some relief from present pain in the muscle.

Physical Changes in Muscles as a Result of Weight Training

A number of important physical changes occur as a result of weight training. First, muscle strength, especially around the joints, increases the efficiency of joint action and helps to prevent injury during physical activity.

Second, strength training also increases the integrity of muscle fibers. For example, individual muscle fibers, which are about the size of a human hair, start to increase in thickness because increased muscle tension is resulting in more protein being deposited in the muscle. There also may be increases in muscle glycogen and energy-rich compounds such as adenosine triphosphate (ATP) and phosphocreatine (PC). Some research indicates that muscle fibers actually split (hyperplasia) as a result of training, but these findings are still highly controversial.

One final physical change that results from weight training is that you look a lot better. Muscle training increases your proportion of fat-free muscles and thereby enhances your aesthetic appearance.

Red and White Muscle Fibers (Endurance and Strength)

Human muscles contain three types of muscle fibers: a slow-twitch type I **red fiber** and two types of fast-twitch type II **white fibers.** Each fiber type is structurally and chemically equipped to perform work for long or short periods of time. For example, fast-twitch fibers are preferentially used for short-term, high-intensity exercise (such as sprinting), while slow-twitch fibers are used during longer, less-intensive exercise (such as long-distance running).

Exercise cannot change the types and numbers of fibers in your muscles since this determination is inherited. However, the efficiency of both red and white muscle fibers can be increased through proper training methods. A specific type of exercise must be used to improve the efficiency of a given fiber type. For example, to increase the metabolic potential of fast-twitch fibers, high-intensity exercise must be used with low repetition. Conversely, exercises of longer duration with lower intensities increase the metabolic potential of slow-twitch fibers. This is one reason why the training sessions of most athletes closely resemble the actual competition. For example, the training of marathon runners primarily involves continuous running, while the training of football players primarily involves shorter running intervals that are interrupted by rest and recovery periods. Research indicates that successful performers in aerobic activities, such as marathon runners, generally have a higher percentage of red fibers and that those engaged in anaerobic events, such as sprinters, have a higher percentage of white fibers. The higher percentages are believed to result from a process of selectivity made by the demands of the activity rather than training. Evidence also indicates that individuals engaged in simultaneous programs of strength and endurance training may have more difficulty gaining strength than those engaged only in a strength program.

Female Muscle Response to Weight Training

Research indicates that, when a woman engages in rigorous weight training, her muscles do not respond in the same way as a man's. Women who use the same weight-training techniques and who work to the same weight capacity as men evidence gains in strength and endurance, but the degree of muscle hypertrophy (the increase in muscle size) is smaller than it is in men. The explanation for this is that women's levels of testosterone (a hormone important in building muscle tissue) are twenty to thirty times less than men. Thus, women do not have to fear that they will develop bulky muscles from weight training. They will increase their strength and endurance, but they will not develop the degree of muscle definition that men do.

Research also has shown that women who engage in weight-training programs tend to lose body fat but maintain their weight because of small gains in lean muscle. This loss in subcutaneous fat may give their muscles increased definition.

Strength and Endurance Training Equipment

A variety of strength and endurance training equipment is available:

1. **Free Weights** Barbells and dumbbells provide exercise to produce both positive and negative phases of muscle contraction.
2. **Universal Gym** This device is designed mainly to duplicate most free-weight exercises. It provides variable resistance in both positive and negative phases of muscle contraction.
3. **Nautilus** This device provides single muscle group training through the full range of movement with variable resistance in both positive and negative phases of muscle contraction.
4. **Cam II** This device provides variable resistance with air pressure generated by a central compressor. Specific muscle groups can be trained together or bilaterally through a full range of movement in both positive and negative phases of muscle contraction.
5. **Polaris** With this device, the weight to be moved is drawn over an oval-shaped plate. Muscles can move through a full range of movement in both positive and negative phases of muscle contraction.
6. **Hydra-Fitness and Eagle Performance** These two methods combine both isokinetic and isotonic principles. The equipment automatically adjusts to the strength and speed of the individual.
7. **Mini-Gym** This device provides for accommodating resistance or isokinetic contraction. The resistance is directly related to the force applied. Variable resistance is provided throughout the entire range of movement.
8. **Exer-Genie** This device allows for both isometric and isotonic movement. A cylinder controls the amount of resistance in a braided nylon line.

When using free weights and nautilus equipment, the following guidelines are important:

1. Use spotters when executing bench presses and squats with free weights.
2. Wear rubber-soled shoes for proper traction.
3. Make sure that metal weights are secured by collars.
4. Chalk your hands with carbonate of magnesium when using free weights.

Periodization of Strength Training—
A New Approach for Athletes

The majority of high-level athletes strength train approximately three to four days a week during the period of strength building and one to three days a week during competition periods. Major lifts, such as pulls and squats, seldom are executed more than two days per week to help prevent the possibility of injury and subsequent reduced performance.

Recently, however, Soviet athletes have developed a unique cyclic training program, called **periodization,** that prepares athletes for maximum performance during peak cycles. Periodization involves four training cycles of different intensities: the load cycle, the recovery cycle, the peak cycle, and the conditioning cycle.

Load Cycle

The load cycle consists of a high number of sets (five to seven) and a moderate number of repetitions (four to seven) at 80 percent of repetition maximum. Within each load cycle are microcycles of about two weeks duration that consist of an intensity progression of heavy to light to moderate work loads. Then the microcycle is repeated using more weight.

The load cycle usually is used during the off-season, in the precompetition period for building strength. This cycle should not be practiced for more than two to three months because of its exhausting nature.

Recovery Cycle

The recovery cycle is a transition period of active rest that separates the strength-building period (load cycle) from the competitive period (peak cycle). The cycle consists of a low to moderate number of sets and repetitions at light to moderate intensity. This cycle generally lasts for two to three weeks.

Peak Cycle

The peak cycle is aimed at producing maximum strength while at the same time allowing for skilled movement. A low number of sets and repetitions and high resistance (80 to 100 percent of repetition maximum) characterize this cycle. Duration is approximately two to three months (equal to that of the load cycle). This cycle is utilized during or immediately preceding competition. Also, like the load cycle, it consists of microcycles that last two to three weeks, during which time maximum resistance is employed only once.

Table 7.4 Example of Muscle Strength Circuit

Station	Exercise	Alloted task time	Pretest repetitions	One-half of pretest repetitions
1	Vertical jumps	60 sec	40	20
2	Push-ups	30 sec	10	5
3	Arm curl	30 sec	15	8
4	Leg press	60 sec	20	10
5	Back hyperextension	60 sec	10	5
6	Upright rowing	60 sec	4	2
7	Bent-knee sit-up	45 sec	12	6
8	Bench press	30 sec	6	3
9	Leg curl	45 sec	8	4
10	Standing overhead press	30 sec	8	4
	Total circuit time	7½ min × 3 = 22½ min		

Conditioning Cycle

The conditioning cycle is a period of active rest following a competitive season. The cycle consists of a moderate number of sets (four to six) and repetitions (eight to ten) at low intensity (60 to 70 percent of repetition maximum). Approximately every three weeks, a slightly higher intensity is employed to maintain strength. The conditioning cycle prevents deconditioning and allows for a mental and physical break from training.

Circuit Training for Weight-Resistance Programs

Circuit training involves a combination of strength and endurance exercises performed in sequence at various stations. This extremely efficient technique can be specifically designed for a variety of different sports activities. For example, the circuit can emphasize strength activities, cardiovascular activities, or a combination of the two.

The circuit should consist of between eight to fifteen stations, with a total circuit completion time of five to twenty minutes. The circuit may be performed more than once during each training session, and you should allow for as many repetitions as possible during the time allotted at each station.

Table 7.4 presents an example of a muscle strength circuit. In this example, ten stations have been selected. The activity at each station depends upon the purpose of the circuit, in this case, building muscle strength. Each task time is set between thirty and sixty seconds. A pretest establishes standards for the circuit. During the pretest, as many repetitions as possible are completed during the allotted task time, with a short period of recovery allowed after each task. The number of repetitions for each circuit task then is determined by taking one-half of those completed in the pretest. The overall circuit time is determined by adding the total time allowed for each task and multiplying by three.

When developing a circuit, try to make the strength exercises as specific as possible to those used in the particular sport for which you are training. Also, for each weight-resistant task in your circuit, periodically increase the intensity to ensure overload. Another important guideline is to separate tasks so that two consecutive stations do not include the same muscle group. Finally, remember to monitor your heart rate to maintain your target heart rate training effect level.

Table 7.5 presents an example of a muscle strength and cardiovascular circuit-training program.

Tracking Your Muscle Strength and Endurance

Appendix B at the back of the book provides record sheets for tracking your progress in increasing your muscle strength and endurance (record sheets B-1, B-4, B-5, and B-6). Keeping records of your advances is a great way of maintaining your motivation.

Key Terms

Circuit Training   A combination of strength and endurance exercises performed in sequence at various stations

Eccentric Loading   When the muscle lengthens as it develops tension

Isokinetic Exercise   A contraction in which the muscle contracts maximally at a constant speed over a full range of the joint movement against a variable resistance

Isometric Exercise   A contraction performed against a fixed or immovable resistance, where tension is developed in the muscle but there is no change in the length of the muscle or the angle of the joint

Isotonic Exercise   Exercise against resistance while the load remains constant, with the resistance varying with the angle of the joint

Muscle Soreness   Muscle pain resulting possibly from chemical or physical changes in the muscle tissue

Muscle Strength   The amount of force that can be exerted by a muscle group for one movement or repetition

Muscle Endurance   The ability of a muscle group to maintain a continuous contraction or repetition over a period of time

Overload   Forcing a muscle to contract at maximum or near maximum tension

Periodization   A training program that involves varying degrees of training cycles throughout the year

Table 7.5 Muscle Strength and Cardiovascular Circuit-Training Program

Duration	Ten weeks
Frequency	Three days per week
Circuits/session	Circuit A: 3; Circuit B: 2
Time/circuit	Circuit A: 7½ min; Circuit B: 15 min
Total time/session	Circuit A: 22½ min; Circuit B: 30 min
Load	40 to 55 percent of 1 RM
Repetitions	As many as possible in thirty seconds
Rest	Fifteen seconds between stations

Muscle strength		Cardiovascular	
Circuit A		*Circuit B*	
Station	*Exercise*	*Station*	*Exercise*
1	Bench press	1	Running (440 yd)
2	Bent-knee sit-ups	2	Push-ups or pull-ups
3	Knee (leg) extension	3	Bent-knee sit-ups
4	Pulldown-lat machine	4	Vertical jumps
5	Back hyperextension	5	Standing (overhead) press
6	Standing (overhead) press	6	Bicycling (3 min)
7	Dead lift	7	Hip stretch
8	Arm curl	8	Rope jumping (1 min)
9	Leg curl (knee flexion)	9	Bent-over rowing
10	Upright rowing	10	Hamstring stretch
		11	Upright rowing
		12	Running (660 yd)

Source: *Sports Psychology,* by Edward L. Fox, Copyright © 1979 by Saunders College Publishing/Holt, Rinehart and Winston. Reprinted by permission of CBS College Publishing.

Plyometric Loading When the muscle is loaded suddenly and then forced to stretch before the contraction for movement occurs

Progressive Resistance The progressive increase in load intensity

Red Fiber Slow-twitch muscle fiber physiologically adapted for endurance activity with a high capacity to use oxygen

Specificity The concept that exercises are specific to the type of training performed

Speed Loading When the resistance is moved as rapidly as possible

Valsalva Maneuver Exhalation against a closed epiglottis, which increases pressure in the chest cavity

White Fiber Fast-twitch muscle fiber physiologically adapted for short-term, high-intensity exercise

Competitive Sports and Advanced Fitness

A Word about Competitive Sports

Once you have achieved an advanced level of cardiovascular fitness, you may be tempted to get involved in competitive running, cycling, skiing, swimming, or other competitive sports. This is perfectly understandable and may even increase your motivation. The important point to remember is that you must keep competitive sports in the proper perspective.

Competition is neither inherently good nor bad but simply one type of human behavior. It is good when it stimulates interest and leads to continued participation, gratification, and self-improvement. It is bad when it promotes hostility, anxiety, and dissatisfaction.

It is self-destructive to judge your success in competitive sports solely on your ability to win. Agonizing about losing a match in the local tournament or finishing way back in the pack in the Sunday morning ten-kilometer run leads only to dissatisfaction. Also, all too often we tend to perceive an opponent as an obstacle blocking our goals. In a very real sense, however, an opponent is a fellow competitor who is presenting us with a challenge. Viewed in this context, competition can provide self-fulfillment for both the "loser" and the "winner."

Too many people are concerned only with winning, and they lose sight of many of the important intrinsic benefits that can be derived from competition, such as increases in skill and endurance and the satisfaction derived from meeting new challenges. Set your own standards and create your own criteria for success and failure. Be aware of your uniqueness and the importance of defining the quality of your personal competitive experience. If you emphasize these values instead of focusing only on winning, competition can enrich your life.

Preparing for Competition

One of the most common problems facing the highly fit individual who decides to get involved in such competition as running, skiing, swimming, or bicycling is determining the sequence of training leading up to competition. Generally, in the early part of the training season, increases in volume (frequency and duration) are most important. As the competition season approaches, however, the intensity of the exercise should be increased and the volume should be decreased. As the competition date nears, both the volume and the intensity of the exercise should be reduced. This is sometimes referred to as the **tapering period.** Most runners use a tapering period of between one and two weeks. Swimmers generally use about two to four weeks for the tapering period.

Determining the volume and intensity of exercise during the tapering period is difficult since there has been very little research in this area. Evidence does indicate, however, that glycogen storage is maximized in about one week and that minor injuries, discomfort, and soreness generally clear up in about two weeks. Both of these are good arguments for a one- to two-week tapering period.

Most training regimens, however, are based upon the past experiences of individual athletes and coaches. Individualized training is important, since you are the best judge of how you are responding to exercise. Also, keep a log of the volume and intensity of your training, and think of long-term, not short-term, competitive goals.

Advanced Fitness

In this section, we look at how popular physical activities and sports are rated with regard to the degree of advanced fitness benefits they provide. Methods of achieving and maintaining advanced fitness, such as long-distance running, interval training, and over-distance training, also are examined.

Rating the Physical Fitness Factors of Popular Sports and Activities

What is the best sport for developing advanced physical fitness? Table 8.1 lists popular physical activities and sports and rates them on four health-related physical fitness factors: cardiovascular efficiency, muscle strength and endurance, body composition, and flexibility. Cardiovascular efficiency has been further broken down into anaerobic and aerobic categories. The ratings are based on a scale of one to five, with five indicating that that particular sport or activity requires a high level of the rated physical fitness factor, and with one indicating that that particular sport or activity requires a low level of the rated physical fitness factor.

For example, in table 8.1, aerobic dance requires an aerobic cardiovascular fitness level of five, while archery requires only an aerobic cardiovascular fitness level of one. To participate in aerobic dance, you should be aerobically fit, while for archery, such aerobic fitness is unnecessary. Table 8.1 also rates the entry level of physical fitness necessary for each sport or activity, along with the skill level requirements of the sport or activity.

Obviously, a number of sports activities, such as bowling and archery, do not develop or maintain cardiovascular fitness. Activities that rate four or above in the aerobic category in table 8.1 are good choices for ensuring cardiovascular fitness.

Individual differences with regard to skill level, motivation, strength, endurance, and so on, however, can directly affect the degree of fitness benefits derived from participating in sports activities. For example, an individual with low-level swimming skills may find water polo much more exhausting than a highly skilled swimmer. The same is true of a beginning skier as compared to an expert. The beginner is much less efficient in controlling extraneous muscle movement and in pacing the activity and probably will require much more energy expenditure than the highly skilled performer. Even equally skilled individuals display different levels of aggression and intensity, especially while competing, and thus may derive different degrees of fitness benefits.

Achieving Advanced Fitness

Methods of achieving advanced fitness include long-distance running, interval training, over-distance training, and many other aerobic and anaerobic options.

Long-Distance Running

Long-distance aerobic events can be extremely challenging and satisfying, yet they pose a number of problems not encountered in lower levels of aerobic activity. As you increase your exercise intensity, your heart, muscles, bones, and joint structures are subjected to increased levels of stress, thereby increasing the possibility of injury and disability. Peak physical condition is vital before attempting long-distance aerobic activities.

The distance you decide to run should be determined by your current fitness level and not by your psychological motivation. You should not attempt distances of five to ten kilometers unless you score in the "excellent" to "superior" category on the 1.5-mile run in chapter 3 and also are currently running approximately twenty-five to forty miles a week. You also should be able to cover the competitive distance comfortably during training at a target heart rate level of between 70 and 75 percent. This is important because during actual competition your target heart rate level may go as high as 85 to 95 percent.

Table 8.1 Health-Related Physical Fitness Factors of Popular Physical Activities and Sports (Scale: 1 = Low Level Required; 5 = High Level Required)

	Entry-level fitness	Cardiovascular efficiency	
		Anaerobic	*Aerobic*
Aerobic Dance	2	4	5
Archery	1	1	1
Backpacking	4	4	4
Badminton	3	3	2
Baseball	3	3	1
Basketball	4	5	3
Bicycling	2	4	5
Bowling	1	1	1
Cross-country skiing	5	5	5
Fencing	2	4	3
Football	3	4	2
Golf (walking)	2	3	3
Gymnastics	4	4	2
Ice Hockey	3	5	4
Jogging	3	3	5
Judo	2	3	1
Lacrosse	4	4	5
Paddle tennis	3	4	2
Racquetball	3	4	3
Rope skipping	3	5	5
Rugby	3	4	3
Skating (recreation)	3	3	3
Skiing downhill	3	5	3
Skin diving	4	4	3
Soccer	3	4	5
Softball	2	3	1
Squash	3	5	2
Surfboarding	5	3	3
Swimming	3	4	5
Tennis (recreation)	3	4	4
Track (field events)	3	4	2
Track (long distances)	5	3	5
Track (up to 400 meters)	4	5	3
Volleyball	3	4	2
Water polo	5	4	5
Weight training	3	4	1
Wrestling	3	4	2

Muscle strength	Muscle endurance	Body composition	Flexibility	Skill level required
3	4	4	4	1
2	1	1	3	2
4	4	4	3	2
3	3	3	3	3
3	3	3	4	3
3	5	4	4	4
4	4	4	3	3
2	2	1	3	2
5	5	5	4	4
4	4	4	4	4
5	5	3	3	3
3	3	3	3	4
5	4	3	5	5
4	4	3	4	4
4	5	4	3	2
4	4	3	5	5
4	4	4	4	4
3	3	3	3	3
3	4	3	4	3
4	5	4	3	3
4	3	3	3	3
3	4	3	3	3
4	5	3	4	5
4	4	4	3	4
4	5	4	4	4
3	3	2	3	3
3	4	4	4	3
4	4	3	3	5
4	5	4	4	3
4	4	4	4	4
5	3	3	4	4
4	5	5	3	2
4	5	4	4	3
4	4	3	4	3
4	5	4	4	4
5	4	3	4	3
5	5	3	4	4

The following are some general guidelines for long-distance running:

1. Ten to fifteen minutes of warm-up (stretching, slow jogging) should precede a run, and the run should be followed by at least an eight- to ten-minute cooling-down period.

2. Twenty to twenty-five percent of competitive training should be above the 70 percent target heart rate level.

3. Four to five months of training should precede competitive runs of five to ten kilometers.

4. If you are running between thirty-five and fifty-five miles a week (training for a ten-kilometer competition), one run a week should be six to ten miles in length.

5. Do not try to increase drastically the number of miles you run from one week to the next. Keep increases at approximately 8 to 10 percent per week.

6. Every four to five weeks, reduce your total weekly mileage by approximately 8 to 10 percent and then increase it by 10 percent the following week.

7. Vary your running distance each day.

8. Practice running both uphill, downhill, and on the level to ensure proper conditioning of all leg muscles and reduce the chances of soreness and injury.

9. Two days out of the week should include interval speed work: for five-kilometer races, two to three miles of two-hundred- to three-hundred-yard runs at a speed faster than your competitive pace with two minutes rest recovery between runs; for ten-kilometer races, five to six miles of two-hundred- to three-hundred-yard runs at a speed faster than your competitive pace with two minutes rest recovery between runs.

10. The week before a ten-kilometer race, you should be able to run six to eight miles comfortably with a fast recovery (forty-five minutes to an hour) and no adverse effects the next day.

11. When your body signals that you are overextending yourself or when you experience pain in your muscles or joints, give way to your feelings and don't try to "run through them."

12. Set your own goals and limits. Don't let others dictate your pace or push you into an unnecessary risk zone.

Interval Training

Interval training is used primarily in competitive training programs for such sports as swimming, skiing, basketball, sprinting, and middle-distance running. It involves periods of intense training interspersed with rest periods. During the rest periods, the chemicals, fatigue products of exercise, can be paid off and new sources of energy resupplied to the muscles. For example, a fifteen-hundred-meter runner might run eight repetitive sixty-second four-hundred-meter runs with three-minute resting periods between each.

One advantage of this regimen over distance running is that the athlete can practice specific pacing and intensity skills involved in running fifteen hundred meters. Another advantage is that the intensity of training on the cardiovascular system is much greater than in distance running. Also, interval training stresses the glycogen system, which results in the production of high levels of lactic acid. High levels of lactic acid produce the feelings of discomfort associated with all intensive exercise. As a result, interval-trained athletes are subject to high levels of physiological stress and thus are familiar with this stress and know how to adjust to it when it confronts them during competition.

Table 8.2 presents an eight-week aerobic interval training program for competitive athletes. During the first two weeks of the program, you need to train four days a week; during the remaining six weeks, you train three days a week. The program consists of grouped exercises (sets), a number of exercises per set (repetitions), and resting times between repetitions (relief intervals). For example, table 8.2 indicates that, on Day 1 of the first week, Set 1 should consist of: 4 × 220 at easy (1:3), where 4 is the number of repetitions, 220 is the training distance in yards, the term *easy* refers to running the 220 at an easy pace, and (1:3) indicates the relief interval (rest three times the amount of time it takes you to run 220 yards before running the next 220). In other words, in the first set, you run 220-yard runs at an easy pace. Between each run, you rest three times the amount of time it takes you to run the 220-yard distance.

Starting with the third week of the interval training program, table 8.2 lists suggested times for running the distances and also for the lengths of the relief intervals. For example, table 8.2 indicates that, on Day 1 of the third week, Set 1 should consist of: 2 × 660 at 2:25 (4:30), which translates into running two 660-yard runs, each in two minutes and twenty-five seconds, and resting four minutes and thirty seconds between each run. These are suggested times. Your best judge is your heart rate response to the exercise.

It is very important that you observe two rules when following the interval training program presented in table 8.2:

1. Do not start the next repetition until the heart rate is down to 150 beats per minute.
2. Do not begin the next set until the heart rate is down to approximately 125 beats per minute.

Table 8.2   Aerobic Interval Training Program for Competitive Athletes

Day		First week		Day		Fifth week	
1	Set 1	4 × 220 at easy	(1:3)	1	Set 1	4 × 660 at 2:05	(4:10)
	Set 2	8 × 110 at easy	(1:3)		Set 2	2 × 440 at 1:30	(2:40)
2	Set 1	2 × 440 at easy	(1:3)	2	Set 1	4 × 220 at 0:37	(1:51)
	Set 2	8 × 110 at easy	(1:3)		Set 2	4 × 220 at 0:37	(1:51)
3	Set 1	2 × 440 at easy	(1:3)		Set 3	4 × 220 at 0:37	(1:51)
	Set 2	6 × 220 at easy	(1:3)		Set 4	4 × 220 at 0:37	(1:51)
4	Set 1	1 × 880 at easy		3	Set 1	2 × 880 at 2:55	(2:55)
	Set 2	6 × 220 at easy	(1:3)		Set 2	2 × 440 at 1:30	(2:40)

Day		Second week		Day		Sixth week	
1	Set 1	2 × 880 at easy	(1:3)	1	Set 1	4 × 660 at 2:00	(4:00)
	Set 2	2 × 440 at easy	(1:3)		Set 2	2 × 440 at 1:18	(2:36)
2	Set 1	6 × 440 at easy	(1:3)	2	Set 1	4 × 220 at 0:36	(1:48)
3	Set 1	3 × 880 at easy	(1:3)		Set 2	4 × 220 at 0:36	(1:48)
4	Set 1	1 × 2,640 at easy			Set 3	4 × 220 at 0:36	(1:48)
					Set 4	4 × 220 at 0:36	(1:48)
				3	Set 1	2 × 880 at 2:50	(2:50)
					Set 2	2 × 440 at 1:18	(2:36)

Day		Third week		Day		Seventh week	
1	Set 1	2 × 660 at 2:25	(4:30)	1	Set 1	2 × 880 at 2:45	(2:45)
	Set 2	2 × 440 at 1:20	(2:40)		Set 2	2 × 440 at 1:26	(2:32)
2	Set 1	4 × 220 at 0:38	(1:54)	2	Set 1	4 × 220 at 0:35	(1:45)
	Set 2	4 × 220 at 0:38	(1:54)		Set 2	4 × 220 at 0:35	(1:45)
	Set 3	4 × 220 at 0:38	(1:54)		Set 3	4 × 220 at 0:35	(1:45)
3	Set 1	1 × 880 at 3:00	(3:00)		Set 4	4 × 220 at 0:35	(1:45)
	Set 2	2 × 440 at 1:20	(2:40)	3	Set 1	1 × 1,320 at 4:30	(2:15)
					Set 2	2 × 1,100 at 3:40	(1:50)

Day		Fourth week		Day		Eighth week	
1	Set 1	3 × 660 at 2:10	(4:20)	1	Set 1	2 × 880 at 2:40	(2:40)
	Set 2	3 × 440 at 1:20	(2:40)		Set 2	2 × 440 at 1:16	(2:32)
2	Set 1	4 × 220 at 0:38	(1:54)	2	Set 1	4 × 220 at 0:34	(1:42)
	Set 2	4 × 220 at 0:38	(1:54)		Set 2	4 × 220 at 0:34	(1:42)
	Set 3	4 × 220 at 0:38	(1:54)		Set 3	4 × 220 at 0:34	(1:42)
	Set 4	4 × 220 at 0:38	(1:54)		Set 4	4 × 220 at 0:34	(1:42)
3	Set 1	2 × 880 at 2:55	(2:55)	3	Set 1	1 × 1,320 at 4:24	(2:12)
	Set 2	2 × 440 at 1:20	(2:40)		Set 2	2 × 1,100 at 3:34	(1:47)

Source: From *Sports Physiology* 2/e by Edward L. Fox. Copyright © 1984 by CBS College Publishing. Reprinted by permission.

Over-Distance Training

Over-distance training involves running, skiing, swimming, or bicycling for a longer distance at a slower pace than that intended for competition; for example, a fifteen-hundred-meter competitor might run sixteen hundred meters at a slower time than it takes to run fifteen hundred meters. Over-distance training is effective for building respiratory capacity, but this training technique violates the principle of specificity. It is difficult to develop a sense of pace because the skill, coordination, and intensity needed, for example, to run fifteen hundred meters are not the same as in running sixteen hundred meters.

Other Options for Advanced Fitness

Anaerobic options for advanced fitness include:

1. **Sprint Training** Repeated sprints of fifty to one hundred yards each with complete recovery between each sprint.
2. **Hollow Sprints** Running two sprints with walking or jogging between sprints. For example, sprinting sixty yards, jogging sixty yards, and then walking sixty yards.
3. **Accelerated Sprints** Increasing running speed from a jog to a stride to a run in fifty- to one-hundred-yard segments.

Aerobic options for advanced fitness include:

1. **Continuous, Fast Running** Long-distance running or swimming at a fast pace. For example, an athlete who usually runs one mile might run 1¼ to 1¾ miles.
2. **Continuous, Slow Running** Long-distance running or swimming (two to five times longer than competitive distance) at a slow pace. The training heart rate should be approximately 150 beats per minute.
3. **Jogging** Continuous, slow running over moderate distances.

Options for advanced fitness that are both aerobic and anaerobic include:

1. **Repetition Running** Repeated periods of exercise interspersed with long rest intervals. For example, running half of a race distance at a slower than competitive time.
2. **Speed Play** Alternating fast and slow running over natural terrain. Can include sports skills—for example, dribbling, kicking.

Key Terms

Interval Training   Periods of intense training interspersed with rest periods

Over-Distance Training   Training for a longer distance at a slower pace than that intended for competition

Tapering Period   The period of time prior to competition during which the volume and the intensity of the exercise is reduced

CHAPTER

9

Nutrition and Weight Control

Need for Accurate Nutritional Information

Not many years ago, the subject of nutrition was of little interest to the American public. With recent research showing relationships between diet and such health problems as heart disease, obesity, diabetes, and cancer, however, interest in nutrition and in research on nutrition has surged. Unfortunately, along with this increased interest has come widespread misinformation and new myths about nutrition. It is often difficult to determine the validity of statements made by a number of so-called experts. Currently, there are a number of major nutritional controversies concerning cholesterol, vitamin C, fiber, sugar, food additives, and various diets. As a result, a continuous need to separate fact from fiction and to educate the public exists in this most vital area.

Major Nutritional Constituents

The major nutritional constituents are carbohydrates, fats, protein, minerals, vitamins, and water.

Carbohydrates

Carbohydrates are chemical compounds containing carbon, hydrogen, and oxygen; examples are sugars and starches. Grain products, fruits, sugar, vegetables, and milk are excellent sources of carbohydrates. Carbohydrates are the major energy sources for muscles so that the muscles can do work. When carbohydrates are broken down, they take the form of sugar in the blood and also are supplied to various brain and nervous system tissue. Carbohydrates are stored in the liver and in muscles in a complex form called **glycogen.**

If you take in a large amount of carbohydrates and the carbohydrates are not fully utilized, the excess can be converted into fat and stored in fat tissue. If your carbohydrate intake is very low, fat cannot be used efficiently, and as a result, fatty acids (organic compounds composed of a carbon chain with hydrogens attached and an acid group at one end) form ketone bodies (a condensation product of fat metabolism produced when carbohydrates are not available), making it difficult for the body to maintain a proper balance between acidity and alkalinity. Also, when carbohydrate intake is low, protein is broken down and used for energy, rather than for building tissue and performing other important functions.

Fats

Fats, which belong to a class of compounds called lipids, supply energy, provide essential fatty acids, and promote the absorption of the fat-soluble vitamins A, D, E, and K. Good sources of fats are nuts, meats, and dairy products. The fat that you consume in your diet is carried by the blood to your muscles, where it is used for energy. It also can be stored in fat cells as adipose tissue.

During exercise, both carbohydrates and fats are burned to provide energy for muscle contraction. Generally, fat is the major energy source for moderate physical activity, while carbohydrates usually provide energy during rigorous, exhaustive activity. Highly conditioned individuals participating in endurance-type activities are able to shift to fat metabolism and burn fat, rather than the sugar (glycogen) that is stored in the muscle cells. As a result, greater amounts of the energy required for an activity can be derived from fat than from carbohydrates.

Fatty acids may be saturated or unsaturated. The type of fat you consume is important because **saturated fats** (fatty acids carrying the maximum possible number of hydrogen ions) tend to raise blood cholesterol while **polyunsaturated fats** (fatty acids that lack four or more hydrogen atoms and have two or more double bonds between carbons) lower it.

Protein

Protein regulates body processes and also may be a source of energy, but its main function is the building and repair of tissue. Excellent sources of protein are meat, fish, poultry, dried beans, peas, nuts, milk, cheese, and eggs.

Minerals

Minerals regulate body processes and maintain body tissue. Minerals are found in all foods except sugar, alcohol, and highly refined fats and oils. They are inorganic compounds smaller than vitamins and are found in very simple forms in foods. Some minerals are used as building blocks for such structures as bones and teeth. Calcium, phosphorus, potassium, sodium, iron, and iodine are a few of the more important required minerals.

Vitamins

Vitamins are organic compounds that are needed in only small amounts by the body. They regulate a number of body processes, including the release of energy from food, and also are used in the metabolism of carbohydrates and fats. All foods, except sugar, alcohol, and highly refined fats and oils, contain vitamins.

Vitamins are classified as either water-soluble or fat-soluble. The water-soluble C and B complex vitamins are not stored in the body and therefore must be continuously supplied by the diet. The fat-soluble A, D, E, and K vitamins are stored in the body. As a result, excessive ingestion of fat-soluble vitamins can have toxic effects.

Water

Water transports nutrients, regulates body temperature, participates in chemical reactions, and removes waste materials. Although water is indispensable for survival, its importance as a vital nutritional constituent often is taken for granted. The body may be able to survive for weeks without food under certain circumstances, but it can survive without water for only a few hours, especially in hot climates.

Anaerobic and Aerobic Energy Systems

Sports require a great deal of energy. However, among the many different sports, there is a wide variety in the amounts of energy required and in how fast that energy is needed. Activities such as sprinting and weight lifting require large amounts of energy in a very short time. Other activities, such as long-distance running and swimming, require lower amounts of energy, but the energy must be delivered over a longer period of time.

The body has three basic energy sources during physical exercise. The first two generally are used for anaerobic activities, while the third normally is used for aerobic activities, even though there is some overlapping of the physiological processes.

The first energy source involves two energy-rich compounds—**ATP (adenosine triphosphate** and **PC (phosphocreatine)**—that are stored directly in the muscle tissue. When the muscle is stimulated through exercise, ATP and PC break down and release immediate energy for muscle contraction. Energy from ATP and PC, however, is only available for a brief period because only very small amounts of these compounds are stored in the muscle.

A second energy source during exercise is supported by sugar, which is stored in the muscles in the form of glycogen. When glycogen is broken down, the released energy produces more ATP. However, when glycogen is burned in the absence of oxygen, it gives off an end product called lactic acid, which results in muscle fatigue. For this reason, this energy source is limited to activities that last approximately one to two minutes. If exercise continues beyond this time, the body is required to draw upon oxygen, the third energy source available during exercise.

The oxygen system can utilize both glycogen and fats as fuel for the production of ATP. Lactic acid, along with the accumulation of calcium 2+ (ions) and heat, are major factors in muscle fatigue. However, when oxygen is utilized through a complex process that occurs in the muscle cells, the oxygen prevents the buildup of lactic acid and promotes the resynthesis of ATP for energy. This system is referred to as aerobic (with oxygen) and is used primarily in endurance activities, such as long-distance running, skiing, and swimming.

Weight Control

A major component of physical fitness is body weight. Considerable evidence indicates that **obesity** (a male who has over 20 percent body fat and a female who has over 30 percent body fat) is associated with a number of diseases, such as coronary artery disease, high blood pressure, and diabetes, as well as feelings of insecurity and a lack of self-esteem. Obesity is one of the major health problems in the United States. In fact, over 30 percent of all Americans over forty years of age are overweight.

Causes of Obesity

Recent research advances have sharpened the focus on the causes of obesity, and a number of new theories have been proposed. Two theories that appear to have some merit are the fat cell theory and the set point theory.

The fat cell theory holds that many individuals consume more food than they need during childhood and, as a result, they produce more fat cells (hyperplasia). By the time they reach adolescence, they may have 40 or 50 percent more fat cells than an individual who has not been overeating. The increased number of fat cells makes it much more difficult for them to lose weight as adults and to maintain a proper weight balance. Diet and exercise can reduce the *size* of the fat cells, but the same *number* of fat cells is carried for life. According to the fat cell theory, children should not be allowed to routinely take in additional food, and they should be encouraged to develop good psychological eating habits and to participate daily in rigorous exercise.

The set point theory suggests that the body has a "set point," or a mechanism for stabilizing weight. Within a narrow range, the set point may be affected by such factors as exercise, which lowers the set point, and too many sweets, which raises it. Raising the set point creates a "need" for additional food, resulting in increased body fat. According to this theory, when you attempt to lose weight by dieting, the body tends to view the diet as a threat to the stability of the set point and therefore can make you feel that you need more to eat and also lower the rate at which you burn up food.

Other factors indirectly related to these two theories also may play an important part in weight gain. For example, the loss of fat from an obese person may trigger a mechanism designed to put the fat back, making it more difficult to lose weight. Evidence also indicates that obesity may be related to depression levels and that eating is a way of compensating for a personality problem. The most recent theory—the brown fat theory—holds that some individuals have malfunctioning brown fat, which is less receptive to chemical breakdown than white fat. Because the brown fat resists breakdown, these people lack the ability to lose kilocalories in the form of heat.

Determining Desired Weight Loss

One difficulty that many people have, once they have determined the percentage of body fat that they would like to lose, is how to convert this percentage into pounds. Table 9.1 provides a simple determination method and an example. Use record sheet B–7 in Appendix B at the back of the book if you want to determine your desired weight loss.

Daily Caloric Needs

A **kilocalorie** (often referred to simply as a "calorie") is the amount of energy required to raise one kilogram of water one degree centigrade. Your overall caloric intake depends on your degree of activity, sex, age, and weight. Of your

---

Table 9.1 Converting Desired Percentage of Body Fat Loss into Pounds

---

1. What is your present weight? _____ lbs

2. Determine your percentage of body fat (chapter 3): _____ %

3. Calculate your desired weight loss. For example, let us assume that you weigh 180 pounds, have 20 percent body fat, and would like to reduce your body fat by 10 percent. What is the equivalent in pounds of a loss of 10 percent of body fat?
   Weight = 180 lbs
   Total fat = 20% × 180 = 36 lbs
   Lean body weight = 180 − 36 lbs = 144 lbs
   y = Desired weight   Desired body fat = 10%

$$y - (y \times .10) = 180 - (180 \times .20)$$
$$1.00\,y - .10y = 180 - 36$$
$$.9y = 144$$
$$y = \frac{144}{.9}$$
$$y = 160$$

   Weight loss required = 180 − 160 = 20 lbs

Therefore, if you weigh 180 pounds and have 20 percent body fat, you have to lose approximately 20 pounds to reduce your body fat to 10 percent.

Table 9.2 Daily Caloric Needs (Determined by Multiplying Body Weight in Pounds with the Appropriate Number Relating to Activity Level)

Physical activity	Women	Men
Sedentary	14	16
Moderately active	18	21
Active	22	26

Table 9.3 Mean Heights and Weights and Recommended Energy Intake

Category	Age (years)	Weight (kg)	Weight (lb)	Height (cm)	Height (in)	Energy needs (kcal) (with range)
Infants	0.0–0.5	6	13	60	24	kg × 115 (95–145)
	0.5–1	9	20	71	28	kg × 105 (80–135)
Children	1–3	13	29	90	35	1,300 (900–1,800)
	4–6	20	44	112	44	1,700 (1,300–2,300)
	7–10	28	62	132	52	2,400 (1,650–3,300)
Males	11–14	45	99	157	62	2,700 (2,000–3,700)
	15–18	66	145	176	69	2,800 (2,100–3,900)
	19–22	70	154	177	70	2,900 (2,500–3,300)
	23–50	70	154	178	70	2,700 (2,300–3,100)
	51–75	70	154	178	70	2,400 (2,000–2,800)
	76+	70	154	178	70	2,050 (1,650–2,450)
Females	11–14	46	101	157	62	2,200 (1,500–3,000)
	15–18	55	120	163	64	2,100 (1,200–3,000)
	19–22	55	120	163	64	2,100 (1,700–2,500)
	23–50	55	120	163	64	2,000 (1,600–2,400)
	51–75	55	120	163	64	1,800 (1,400–2,200)
	76+	55	120	163	64	1,600 (1,200–2,000)
Pregnancy	—	—	—	—	—	+300
Lactation	—	—	—	—	—	+500

Source: From *Recommended Dietary Allowances,* revised 1980, reprinted with permission of the National Academy Press, Washington, D.C.

total daily caloric intake, approximately 58 percent should be in the form of carbohydrates, 30 percent in fats, and about 12 percent in protein. If you engage in very rigorous activity (running or playing tennis four or five times a week), you need more calories to meet the demands of the exercise. If you lead a sedentary life, you need fewer calories. If you are putting on weight, you probably are taking in too many calories. If you are losing weight, you are not taking in a sufficient number of calories.

Table 9.2 presents a general idea of daily caloric needs for men and women. Choose your present level of physical activity and multiply the appropriate value by your present weight in pounds to determine your daily caloric needs. Tables 9.3 and 9.4 are more exacting measures of your daily caloric needs.

Table 9.4 Recommended Daily Dietary Allowances (RDA) (Designed for the Maintenance of Good Nutrition of Practically All Healthy Persons in the United States)

Sex-age category	Persons						Food energy	Protein	Minerals			Vita-min A	Thia-min	Ribo-flavin	Nia-cin	Ascorbic acid
	Age		Weight		Height				Cal-cium	Phos-phorus	Iron					
	Years From	To	Kilo-grams	Pounds	Centi-meters	Inches	Calories	Grams	Milli-grams	Milli-grams	Milli-grams	Inter-national units	Milli-grams	Milli-grams	Milli-grams	Milli-grams
Infants	0	0.5	6	13	60	24	kg × 115 lb × 52.3	kg × 2.2 lb × 1.0	360	240	10	1,400	0.3	0.4	6	35
	0.5	1	9	20	71	28	kg × 105 lb × 47.7	kg × 2.0 lb × 0.9	540	360	15	2,000	.5	.6	8	35
Children	1	3	13	29	90	35	1,300	23	800	800	15	2,000	.7	.8	9	45
	4	6	20	44	112	44	1,700	30	800	800	10	2,500	.9	1.0	11	45
	7	10	28	62	132	52	2,400	34	800	800	10	3,300	1.2	1.4	16	45
Males	11	14	45	99	157	62	2,700	45	1,200	1,200	18	5,000	1.4	1.6	18	50
	15	18	66	145	176	69	2,800	56	1,200	1,200	18	5,000	1.4	1.7	18	60
	19	22	70	154	177	70	2,900	56	800	800	10	5,000	1.5	1.7	19	60
	23	50	70	154	178	70	2,700	56	800	800	10	5,000	1.4	1.6	18	60
	51+		70	154	178	70	2,400	56	800	800	10	5,000	1.2	1.4	16	60
Females	11	14	46	101	157	62	2,200	46	1,200	1,200	18	4,000	1.1	1.3	15	50
	15	18	55	120	163	64	2,100	46	1,200	1,200	18	4,000	1.1	1.3	14	60
	19	22	55	120	163	64	2,100	44	800	800	18	4,000	1.1	1.3	14	60
	23	50	55	120	163	64	2,000	44	800	800	18	4,000	1.0	1.2	13	60
	51+		55	120	163	64	1,800	44	800	800	18	4,000	1.0	1.2	13	60
Pregnant							+300	+30	+400	+400	18+	+1,000	+.4	+.3	+2	+20
Lactating							+500	+20	+400	+400	18	+2,000	+.5	+.5	+5	+40

Source: From *Recommended Dietary Allowances*, revised 1980, reprinted with permission of the National Academy Press, Washington, D.C.

Appendix C at the back of the book presents a detailed listing of the caloric content of a variety of foods in the different food groups. Use record sheet B–8 in Appendix B to record your daily caloric intake.

Losing Weight through Exercise

The belief that the best way to lose weight is to go on a diet is a misconception. Fad and crash diets can result in very serious health consequences. Even normal dieting can cause anxiety and depression. Also, repeated weight gains and losses can cause serious problems, such as an increased percentage of fat. An alternative to dieting is losing weight through exercise.

Calories Burned through Physical Activity

Exercise is an integral part of any weight-loss program. However, losing weight through exercise takes time. After all, it has taken many years to put on the extra weight, and you cannot expect to lose it in a matter of several days. Approximately thirty-five hundred calories must be burned to use up one pound of stored fat. If, for example, your food intake in one day is equivalent to twenty-four hundred calories and you burn up twenty-four hundred calories in your everyday activities, you will be in caloric balance—you will not gain or lose weight. If, however, you burn up an additional one hundred calories a day (for a total of twenty-five hundred calories) by jogging or walking a mile, in thirty-five days you probably would lose one pound of fat. If this loss of one hundred extra calories a day was extended for one year, you could lose approximately twelve to thirteen pounds of fat, assuming that you haven't increased your food intake. By increasing your exercise to burn up two hundred calories a day, you could lose almost twenty-four pounds in a year. Combining increased exercise with a decrease in food intake usually increases weight loss. Maximum weight loss a week, however, should not exceed two pounds, or a one thousand calories per day deficit.

The more rigorous or exhausting the physical activity, the greater the number of calories burned per minute. For example, activities like running and cross-country skiing probably burn up the highest number of calories—up to twenty calories per minute! Swimming also rates very high in caloric expenditure.

You can approximate the number of calories you are burning per minute during rigorous activity by monitoring your pulse. Generally, if your pulse rate is about 120 or below, you probably are burning about five calories per minute. If your pulse rate is 120 to 150 beats per minute, you are burning five to ten calories per minute. If your pulse rate is about 150, you probably are burning ten or more calories per minute. For example, if you jog thirty minutes with a pulse rate that averages between 130 and 140, you might burn up to three hundred calories (10 cal $\times$ 30 min) in a half hour.

The speed at which you run is another important factor in caloric expenditure. If you run at 5 miles per hour, your caloric expenditure will be about ten

Table 9.5 Approximate Energy Cost (in Kilocalories) of Various Physical Activities

Sport or activity	Kilocalories expended per minute (kcal/min) of activity
Climbing	10.7–13.2
Cycling 5.5 MPH	4.5
9.4 MPH	7.0
13.1 MPH	11.1
Dancing	3.3–7.7
Football	8.9
Golf	5.0
Gymnastics	
Balancing	2.5
Abdominal exercises	3.0
Trunk bending	3.5
Arm swinging, hopping	6.5
Rowing 51 str/min	4.1
87 str/min	7.0
97 str/min	11.2
Running	
Short distance	13.3–16.6
Cross-country	10.6
Tennis	7.1
Skating (fast)	11.5
Skiing, moderate speed	10.8–15.9
Uphill, maximum speed	18.6
Squash	10.2
Swimming	
Breaststroke	11.0
Backstroke	11.5
Crawl (55 yd/min)	14.0
Wrestling	14.2

Source: Reprinted by permission of the American Alliance for Health, Physical Education, Recreation and Dance, 1900 Association Drive, Reston, Virginia 22091.

calories per minute. If you speed up to about 7.5 miles per hour, you burn about fifteen calories per minute. At 10 miles per hour, you might burn as many as twenty calories per minute, while at 12 miles per hour, you have the potential of using up twenty-five calories per minute.

Tables 9.5 and 9.6 give you a general idea of the number of kilocalories expended per minute during exercise. Tables 9.7–9.10 indicate how much walking, jogging, bicycling, and swimming you must do to burn enough calories to lose weight. Appendix D at the back of the book relates calorie expenditure per minute for a wide variety of activities to body weight. Use record sheet B–9 in Appendix B to keep track of your daily caloric intake and expenditure.

Table 9.6 Typical Criteria for the Classification of Exercise Intensity

Exercise intensity classification	Criteria heart rate	Energy expenditure (kcal/hr)	Perceived exertion
Very light	<110	<110	Very, very easy
Light	110–120	111–270	Easy, no pain or discomfort
Moderate	121–150	270–400	Somewhat difficult and slight discomfort
Heavy	151–160	401–550	Difficult, uncomfortable, and some pain
Very heavy	161–180	550–669	Very difficult and painful
Exhaustive	>180	>700	Extremely difficult and painful

Source: From Hage, Phillip, "Perceived Exertion: One Measure of Exercise Intensity," in *The Physician and Sports Medicine,* September 1981, pp. 136–46. © 1981 McGraw-Hill Healthcare Group. Reprinted by permission.

Table 9.7 Days Required to Lose Five to Twenty-Five Pounds by Walking* and Lowering Daily Calorie Intake

Minutes of walking	+	Reduction of calories per day (in kcal)	Days to lose 5 pounds	Days to lose 10 pounds	Days to lose 15 pounds	Days to lose 20 pounds	Days to lose 25 pounds
30		400	27	54	81	108	135
30		600	20	40	60	80	100
30		800	16	32	48	64	80
30		1,000	13	26	39	52	65
45		400	23	46	69	92	115
45		600	18	36	54	72	90
45		800	14	28	42	56	70
45		1,000	12	24	36	48	60
60		400	21	42	63	84	105
60		600	16	32	48	64	80
60		800	13	26	39	52	65
60		1,000	11	22	33	44	55

Source: From *Exercise Equivalents of Foods: A Practical Guide for the Overweight,* by Frank Konishi. Copyright © 1983 by Southern Illinois University Press. Reprinted with permission of the publisher.
*Walking briskly (3.5 to 4 MPH), calculated at 5.2 cal/min.

Table 9.8 Days Required to Lose Five to Twenty-Five Pounds by Jogging* and Lowering Daily Calorie Intake

Minutes of jogging +	Reduction of calories per day (in kcal)	Days to lose 5 pounds	Days to lose 10 pounds	Days to lose 15 pounds	Days to lose 20 pounds	Days to lose 25 pounds
30	400	21	42	63	84	105
30	600	17	34	51	68	85
30	800	14	28	42	56	70
30	1,000	12	24	36	48	60
45	400	18	36	54	72	90
45	600	14	28	42	56	70
45	800	12	24	36	48	60
45	1,000	10	20	30	40	50
60	400	15	30	45	60	75
60	600	12	24	36	48	60
60	800	11	22	33	44	55
60	1,000	9	18	27	36	45

Source: From *Exercise Equivalents of Foods: A Practical Guide for the Overweight*, by Frank Konishi. Copyright © 1983 by Southern Illinois University Press. Reprinted with permission of the publisher.
*Alternate jogging and walking, calculated at 10 cal/min.

Table 9.9 Days Required to Lose Five to Twenty-Five Pounds by Bicycling* and Lowering Daily Calorie Intake

Minutes of bicycling +	Reduction of calories per day (in kcal)	Days to lose 5 pounds	Days to lose 10 pounds	Days to lose 15 pounds	Days to lose 20 pounds	Days to lose 25 pounds
30	400	25	50	75	100	125
30	600	19	38	57	76	95
30	800	17	34	51	68	85
30	1,000	13	26	39	52	65
45	400	22	44	66	88	110
45	600	17	34	51	68	85
45	800	14	28	42	56	70
45	1,000	12	24	36	48	60
60	400	19	38	57	76	95
60	600	15	30	45	60	75
60	800	13	26	39	52	65
60	1,000	11	22	33	44	55

Source: From *Exercise Equivalents of Foods: A Practical Guide for the Overweight*, by Frank Konishi. Copyright © 1983 by Southern Illinois University Press. Reprinted with permission of the publisher.
*Bicycling at approximately 7 MPH, calculated at 6.5 cal/min.

Table 9.10 Days Required to Lose Five to Twenty-Five Pounds by Swimming* and Lowering Daily Calorie Intake

Minutes of swimming	+	Reduction of calories per day (in kcal)	Days to lose 5 pounds	Days to lose 10 pounds	Days to lose 15 pounds	Days to lose 20 pounds	Days to lose 25 pounds
30		400	23	46	69	92	115
30		600	18	36	52	72	90
30		800	14	28	42	56	70
30		1,000	12	24	36	48	60
45		400	19	38	57	76	95
45		600	15	30	45	60	75
45		800	13	26	39	52	65
45		1,000	11	22	33	44	55
60		400	16	32	48	64	80
60		600	14	28	42	56	70
60		800	11	22	33	44	55
60		1,000	10	20	30	40	50

Source: From *Exercise Equivalents of Foods: A Practical Guide for the Overweight,* by Frank Konishi. Copyright © 1983 by Southern Illinois University Press. Reprinted with permission of the publisher.
*Swimming at about thirty yards per minute, calculated at 8.5 cal/min.

Losing Fat

Exercise affects your body's ability to utilize fat in a number of ways. For example, the amount of fat lost due to exercise generally is proportional to the intensity and duration of the exercise. The body tends to shift from burning fat during moderate activities to burning stored carbohydrates (glycogen) during very rigorous activities. Therefore, at very high levels of exercise, when the amount of oxygen is limited, carbohydrates are burned in preference to fat. During moderate physical activity, such as jogging, which can be continued for a much longer period of time, fat is the main source of energy. Even though you burn fewer calories per unit of time during moderate exercise as compared to rigorous exercise, you are able to continue exercising for a much longer period, thus producing a greater overall caloric expenditure of fat.

As mentioned before, while the number of fat cells does not decrease as a result of exercise, their size can be substantially reduced through diet and exercise. Also, blood flow through stored fat increases during exercise, which aids in the transport of fat to working muscles. An interesting corollary is that research indicates that high levels of lactic acid can interfere with fat breakdown. Thus, individuals in good physical condition, who do not usually accumulate as high a level of lactic acid as those who are not as physically fit, can continue exercising for much longer periods of time before lactic acid accumulates and interferes with fat breakdown.

Increased Caloric Expenditure after Exercise

The increased metabolism brought about by rigorous physical exercise can persist for a number of hours after the exercise has ceased and may even enable you to burn up more fat. For example, while jogging a half hour, you may burn around ten calories a minute for a total of three hundred calories. After you stop jogging, instead of returning to preexercise levels, your body may continue burning ten calories a minute for an hour or more. Therefore, it is not only during exercise that you increase metabolic activity, but also afterwards—until the body has paid off the debt incurred while exercising.

How to Gain Weight

If you want to gain weight in a hurry and it does not matter to you if the additional weight is in muscle or fat, you can add any kind of calories to achieve the desired gain. Fatty foods have more calories than protein or carbohydrates per weight; therefore, you can gain weight more quickly and easily with a high-fat diet. Eating fat to gain weight, however, can increase the possibility of nutrition-related diseases, such as coronary heart disease.

The best way to gain weight is to build yourself up through very careful and consistent physical training. Eat a well-balanced nutritious diet with enough calories in the form of complex carbohydrates to support a weight gain. Table 9.11 presents an example of a high-calorie diet.

Eating and Exercise

Before rigorous exercise, you should be careful about not only *what* you eat but also *when* you eat it. Your diet and your meal-timing could affect your performance.

Digestion and Rigorous Exercise

There are a number of reasons why you should avoid eating just prior to rigorous exercise. First, when you go from rest to exercise, a large amount of blood is shifted away from the stomach and intestines to other exercising muscles. Therefore, if you have food in your stomach and intestines during exercise, there will be insufficient blood to digest the food properly and you may experience digestive distress, such as nausea and vomiting. Second, rigorous exercise reduces gastric juice secretion, which plays a major role in breaking down food for digestion. Third, lactic acid levels increase during exercise, which can affect the ability of the stomach to break down food. Fourth, even light exercise has been shown to negatively affect digestion in the small intestines. Finally, the feeling of fullness

Table 9.11 High-Calorie Diet—Six Thousand Calories in Six Meals

Breakfast	Snack	Dinner	Snack

1/2 cup orange juice
1 cup oatmeal
1 cup lowfat milk
1 scrambled egg
1 slice whole-wheat
  toast
1½ teaspoons
  margarine
1 tablespoon jam
 	
Total calories: 665
	1 peanut butter
	  sandwich
	1 banana
	1 cup grape juice
	
	Total calories: 485
		1 cup cream of
		  mushroom soup
		2 pieces oven-
		  baked chicken
		1 candied sweet
		  potato
		1 dinner roll and
		  margarine
		1 cup carrots and
		  peas
		1/2 cup coleslaw
		1 piece cherry pie
		1 beverage
		
		Total calories: 1,615
			1 cup cashew nuts
			1 cup cocoa
			
			Total calories: 1,045

Lunch	Snack		

5 fish sticks with
  tartar sauce
1 large serving,
  French fries
1 green salad with
  avocado and
  French dressing
1 cup lemon sherbet
2 granola cookies
1 cup lowfat milk
 	
Total calories: 1,505
	1 cup mixed dried
	  fruit
	1½ cups malted
	  milk
	
	Total calories: 660
			Daily total calories:
			  5,975

Source: High Caloric Diet Table, *Food For Sport*, by N. J. Smith, Copyright 1976, Bull Publishing. Palo Alto, CA.

after eating may have a psychological effect on your performance during rigorous exercise. All of these factors are good arguments for allowing at least four hours to pass between a heavy meal and rigorous exercise.

As an example of how food and digestion can affect rigorous exercise, let us consider the precompetition eating regimen you would follow if you were a long-distance runner.

For long-distance competitive running, carbohydrates are your main source of energy, and it is therefore imperative that you have a sufficient amount of carbohydrates available before you run. If you are going to compete on a Saturday, for example, you should undergo only a moderate workout on Thursday and a light workout on Friday. This prevents you from depleting your stored glycogen. Your prerunning meal should be fairly light and at least four hours before you run. The two meals preceding your prerunning meal should be high in carbohydrates, such as oatmeal, toast, jam, and honey.

Before a competitive run, keep the following eating guidelines in mind:

1. Avoid foods that are distasteful to you and that you simply don't enjoy eating. They could have a negative psychological effect on your performance.
2. Avoid spicy foods and roughage that might irritate your gastrointestinal tract.
3. Avoid fatty foods for at least four hours before competition since they can slow down your digestive process.
4. Carbohydrates can be eaten two hours before competition with generally no problems.
5. On very hot days, drink some water thirty minutes before the competition.
6. Keep your protein foods to a minimum because an excess of protein may cause an increase of acidosis in the blood, which may increase your chances of fatigue.
7. Derive your fluids from soups, such as bouillon, and fruit juices.

High-Energy Foods for Rigorous Exercise

Considerable evidence indicates that all of us should increase the proportion of complex carbohydrates in our diets while reducing the percentages of fats and proteins. Good sources of complex carbohydrates are brown rice, whole-wheat breads, oatmeal, beans, peas, potatoes, pasta, and a number of fresh fruits and vegetables. Complex carbohydrates are especially important for those individuals involved in rigorous exercise requiring high levels of energy expenditure. When carbohydrates are broken down, they produce high levels of energy with relatively small amounts of harmful waste products. If you consume excessive amounts of fats and protein, your body becomes overloaded with their toxic by-products of metabolism, which may result in decreased physical performance. For example, excessive amounts of protein (over 15 percent of daily diet or in excess of eighty-five to ninety grams) results in increased mineral and water loss and acidosis (excessive acid in blood and body fluids).

Table 9.12 shows current and recommended nutritional allowances, as well as nutritional allowances recommended for the high-energy needs of rigorous physical exercise.

Caffeine and Exercise

A number of individuals are experimenting with the use of caffeine as a means of delaying fatigue during rigorous activity. This use is based on some recent evidence that indicates that caffeine may enable the body to more efficiently utilize fatty acids for energy production. The studies in this area, however, are fairly limited and should be viewed with caution.

Table 9.12 Current, Recommended, and High-Energy Nutritional Allowances

	Current	Recommended by American Heart Association	Recommended for high-energy needs
Fats	42%	30%	10 to 20%
Protein	12%	12%	10 to 12%
Complex carbohydrates	22%	48%	60 to 80%
Sugar	24%	10%	5 to 10%

It is important to remember that caffeine is a stimulant. Large amounts of caffeine can have a variety of effects on the body, such as increased urine output, constriction in the circulatory system, and stimulation of the heart (which may result in irregular heartbeats). Also, recent research has associated frequent coffee drinking in middle-aged men with high levels of cholesterol and low-density lipoprotein, which are associated with a greater risk of coronary heart disease. (One cup of coffee may contain approximately 100 to 150 milligrams of caffeine; tea contains a little less.)

Special Diets

Special diets have been suggested for all kinds of reasons—for losing weight, for increasing physical well-being, and for improving physical performance. Some of these diets are fads and are potentially dangerous. The others must be undertaken cautiously and only with complete knowledge of what is required to meet all daily nutritional requirements and to avoid any of the diet's possible side effects.

Fad Diets

A number of fad diets with varying combinations of nutrients unfortunately have found wide acceptance because of media misinformation and public ignorance. Be very wary of these diets because they may have a number of dangerous consequences. For example, individuals on diets that do not allow for protein or that are low in protein may suffer a loss of muscle tissue and severe weakness. A high-fat diet, sometimes advocated in combination with high protein and very little carbohydrates, may produce a loss of nutrients and electrolytes, very high cholesterol levels, and diarrhea. A high-protein and high-fat diet with low carbohydrates may produce kidney problems, dizziness, weakness, dehydration, irritability, and uric acid formation. Low-fat diets may lead to dry skin, constipation, irritability, stiff joints, and a number of other problems.

Other fad diets that have enjoyed unwarranted popularity include the low-carbohydrate diet, "super-protein" diets, and vitamin and mineral supplemental diets. "Diet foods" and using drugs to lose weight also are discussed in this section.

Low-Carbohydrate Diet

The oldest and the most popular reducing diet is the low-carbohydrate diet. Although it is currently being advertised as new and revolutionary, it actually is a very old regimen that resurfaces every few years, generally under a new name. A low-carbohydrate diet involves cutting your carbohydrate intake to around sixty grams a day or less, while eating all of the protein and fatty foods that you want.

As you might suspect, there are a number of problems with the low-carbohydrate method of losing weight. The major indictment of the diet is that it is dangerous. Even though some physicians still prescribe this diet, a majority of the medical profession do not consider it medically safe. While restricting carbohydrates in the diet can sometimes produce a dramatic weight loss, no experimental evidence indicates that fat loss occurs if the dieter consumes more calories than he or she is expending, as can happen with the low-carbohydrate diet. Also, whatever fat loss *does* occur as a result of a low-carbohydrate diet appears to come from the toxic effects of ketones (end products of fat breakdown), which produce nausea and thus suppress the appetite. These ketone bodies can cause severe injury to the body tissue, in particular to the blood vessels. The low-carbohydrate diet also can produce weight loss because of a loss of salt. Since water follows salt, much of the weight loss seen on the bathroom scale may be due to the excretion of salt and water. It is dangerous to upset the water and electrolyte balance, and this "weight loss" will be regained as soon as the dieter reumes a carbohydrate diet. The low-carbohydrate diet's high fat content also tends to contribute to atherosclerosis.

"Super-Protein" Diets

Some athletes ingest large amounts of protein supplements, believing that doing so will help them to build up their muscles and energy level, even though there is no scientific justification for the use of these supplements. Athletes generally do not need additional protein but additional calories in the form of complex carbohydrates to provide energy for muscle activity. Most athletes already consume twice as much protein as they can possibly use and probably are wasting about half as much as they eat.

It is impossible to force extra amounts of protein into the muscles just by eating more. For muscle cells to accept additional protein, additional demands have to be made upon the muscles. To make a muscle grow, you have to overload it. The muscle generally responds by taking in more nutrients and subsequently accelerating its growth.

The so-called "super-protein" diets are unnecessary, expensive, and in some cases harmful. For example, with large amounts of protein, the blood level of uric acid may increase and damage the kidneys and make the joints more susceptible to injuries. As for energy derived from protein, you burn up as much protein reading a book as running a track at top speed. The body burns protein for energy only in starvation.

Vitamin and Mineral Supplemented Diets

Supplementing your diet with vitamins and minerals above the minimum daily requirement does not improve physical performance. In fact, excessive intake of vitamins A, D, and K can cause toxic effects. Minimum daily vitamin and mineral requirements are met easily through a normal, well-balanced diet.

The one exception to this may be the iron requirement of females engaged in rigorous physical activity, particularly after menstrual blood loss. These women have been found to have significantly decreased levels of iron in their blood. Since overdoses of iron can be toxic, however, these women should take iron supplements only after consulting with a physician.

One vitamin in particular—vitamin E—has been promoted as a cure-all. At the present time, however, there is no evidence to indicate that vitamin E enhances an individual's ability to perform rigorous work. There also is no evidence that it reduces heart disease, increases sex drive, lengthens life span, reduces infection, or improves your complexion. Vitamin E is a fat-soluble vitamin (which means that it can be stored in the body) and is important for the prevention of some blood disorders and for the excretion of creatine. It is found in such foods as beans, fruits, vegetables, whole grains, margarines, and oils. Deficiencies in vitamin E are extremely rare.

"Diet Foods"

A common food myth is that certain kinds of foods burn up stored fat and play a part in weight reduction. All foods contain calories; therefore, no foods can serve as weight reducers. Grapefruit and the other substances around which this myth flourishes, such as safflower oil, vinegar, vitamin B6, and lecithin, have no effect whatsoever on fat loss. Substances that are referred to as "diet foods," such as diet bread, diet cookies, and diet beer, all contain calories, and if you consume enough of them, you will gain weight.

Using Drugs to Lose Weight

A number of prescription drugs, such as amphetamines and barbiturates, have been used as diet aids to reduce appetite. These drugs, however, have many dangerous side effects and really don't get at the overweight individual's major problem—changing his or her eating pattern. No over-the-counter drugs are effective in reducing fat or appetite. The so-called bulk reducers, such as glucomanan, have little effect on the appetite; neither do other so-called appetite depressants, such as propradine.

Vegetarian Diets

For years, Americans have had a love affair with meat. Recently, however, for a variety of reasons, many individuals have decided to reduce and in some cases eliminate meat from their diet. There are many degrees of meat exclusion among vegetarians. Individuals who exclude all foods of animal origin and eat only raw fruits, seeds, and nuts are called pure vegetarians. Individuals who include milk, eggs, and cheese, as well as vegetables, fruits, and grains in their diet are called ovo-lacto vegetarians. Other individuals modify these vegetarian diets to suit their own beliefs.

There are a number of important health considerations related to a vegetarian diet. For example, ovo-lacto or pure vegetarians generally have a lower serum cholesterol count and reduced heart disease, as well as a lower incidence of certain types of cancer. The reduced heart disease may be the result of the lower fat and cholesterol intake. The higher fiber intake of the vegetarian may offer some protection against cancer of the colon. In addition, individuals on vegetarian diets tend to have a greater bone density in older age and fewer incidents of osteoporosis, a disease that degenerates the bones.

As with any kind of diet, the more foods or types of foods that are excluded, the more likely that a nutritional deficiency will occur. The main concern with a vegetarian diet is ensuring sufficient amounts of daily protein. Most research indicates that vegetarians consume enough foods to meet their energy needs and also their protein requirements. A pure vegetarian diet that meets all nutritional needs, however, is generally fairly high in bulk, and this makes it sometimes difficult to take in enough food to meet the energy needs required for rigorous physical activity.

A common problem for those on a vegetarian diet is the selection of foods with a high concentration of iron. Iron is important for the production of hemoglobin and the red blood cells that carry oxygen. Individuals with low hemoglobin and a low red cell count may find it difficult to engage in very rigorous exercise and may fatigue easily. Vegetarians must also be cautious in their selection of iron- and zinc-rich foods or alternative foods because iron and zinc are not well absorbed from vegetable foods.

Fasting

The main source of energy for your exercise comes from your diet. In essence, when you eat, you refuel. When you don't eat, or **fast,** your body is forced to find other sources of energy and draws upon stored reserves of carbohydrates and fats and eventually upon muscle tissue. Glucose in the blood is quickly used up. The body then draws upon glycogen in the muscles. When the glycogen is burned up, the body depends on fatty acids as an energy source. The problem here is that brain cells cannot depend upon fatty acids for fuel—they need glucose since glucose is the only nutrient that can get through their membranes. When glucose is not available, brain cells find another source of glucose in the form of amino acids that can be converted to glucose. These amino acids are found only in complete protein that is stored in the muscle tissue. Thus, the muscle tissue is broken down to provide energy. As a fast continues, the energy output of the body is sharply reduced and the muscles shrink in mass and have less energy to work.

Fasting also causes the body to produce ketones, which are a combination of fatty acids that normally are found only in small amounts in the body. During fasting, however, very large numbers of ketones are produced and may spill over into the urine, resulting in a serious health condition known as ketosis.

Carbohydrate Loading

Carbohydrate loading involves increasing the amount of glycogen stored by the skeletal muscles through special diets and exercise. The average individual stores approximately fifteen grams of glycogen for each kilogram of muscle weight.

There are three different methods of carbohydrate loading. In the first, you consume a high-carbohydrate diet for three or four days, after several days of a normal, mixed diet. This technique can increase the amount of stored glycogen by 30 percent.

A second procedure for carbohydrate loading combines exercise and diet. The muscles that you want to load with carbohydrates are first exhausted of their glycogen storage through rigorous exercise. Then, you follow a high-carbohydrate diet for several days. This routine has been shown to double glycogen storage.

The third method of carbohydrate loading involves exercise and two special diets. Once again, exercise is used to induce glycogen depletion. This is followed by a three-day diet that is very low in carbohydrates and high in fats and protein. After this, you consume a diet high in carbohydrates for three additional days. Exhausting exercise may be performed during the days of the high-fat and high-protein diet but not during the high-carbohydrate diet. This last procedure has been shown to increase glycogen storage as much as four times the amount normally stored in the muscle.

Carbohydrate loading is not without its side effects, however, especially when a high-protein, low-carbohydrate diet is combined with exercise. For example, carbohydrate loading can result in a feeling of stiffness and heaviness from the additional glycogen that has been loaded in the muscle. Also, current evidence indicates that carbohydrate loading may cause kidney malfunctioning that results in myoglobin in the urine. In addition, athletes who persist in carbohydrate loading may experience chest pain and some electrocardiographic changes similar to those observed in patients with heart disease. These side effects could be very serious and require immediate medical attention.

Table 9.13 Basic Nutritional Guidelines

1. Eat a variety of foods.
2. Maintain your ideal weight.
3. Avoid too much fat.
4. Consume a maximum of three hundred milligrams of cholesterol a day (the equivalent of one egg).
5. Avoid too much sugar.
6. Avoid too much sodium.
7. Eat complex carbohydrates, starch, and fiber.

Source: *Nutrition and your heart: Dieting guidelines for Americans.* U.S. Department of Health and Human Services.

Age and Diet

For each subsequent decade after the age of twenty-five, the body's ability to metabolize food slows down about 4 percent. Thus, if your diet remains unchanged as you get older, you are likely to gain weight because you are not burning up your food as efficiently. One way to counteract this problem is to increase your daily exercise to burn up the extra calories. Another, of course, is to decrease the amount of food that you consume.

As you get older, it also is likely that even if you maintain the same body weight, your percentage of body fat may increase. Over the years, lean muscle tissue can be replaced by increased fat deposits. Again, daily exercise can help to prevent this.

The quantity of essential nutrients in your diet also should be carefully regulated as you age. Protein should constitute about 12 percent of the calories in your diet. No more than 20 percent of your calories should come from fats, with the remainder coming from carbohydrates. While the need for protein is the same for adults as it is for young people, adults have to get their protein from less food to avoid gaining weight. Limiting your fat intake should help you to cut calories and to stop the development of atherosclerosis. Also, excessive fats interfere with calcium absorption and promote osteoporosis (bone degeneration). Your vitamins and minerals can be obtained from protein sources and foods high in complex carbohydrates, such as fruits, vegetables, and grains, rather than from fats. Such minerals as calcium and iron are very important in your diet as you age to maintain your hemoglobin since low levels of hemoglobin can result in fatigue and apathy.

Table 9.13 presents basic nutritional guidelines from the U.S. Department of Health and Human Services, while table 9.14 offers three example menus for different levels of calorie intake.

Table 9.14 Calorie Countdown Menus

1,200 Calories	1,800 Calories	2,400 Calories
Breakfast		
Orange juice, ½ cup	Orange juice, ¾ cup	Orange juice, 1 cup
Bran flakes with raisins, ½ cup	Bran flakes with raisins, ½ cup	Bran flakes with raisins, ½ cup
Milk, whole, ½ cup	Milk, whole, ½ cup	Milk, whole, ½ cup
Whole-wheat toast, 1 slice	Whole-wheat toast, 1 slice	Whole-wheat toast, 1 slice
Coffee/tea	Jelly, 2 teaspoons	Jelly, 1 tablespoon
	Coffee/tea	Coffee/tea
Lunch		
Sandwich:	Sandwich:	Sandwich:
Ham, 2 ounces	Ham, 2 ounces	Ham, 2 ounces
Cheese, 1 slice (1 ounce)	Cheese, 1 slice (1 ounce)	Cheese, 1 slice (1 ounce)
Lettuce	Lettuce	Lettuce
Tomato, ½ medium	Tomato, ½ medium	Tomato, ½ medium
Enriched bread, 2 slices	Enriched bread, 2 slices	Enriched bread, 2 slices
Apple, 1 medium	Salad dressing, 2 teaspoons	Salad dressing, 2 teaspoons
Coffee/tea	Apple, 1 medium	Apple, 1 medium
	Coffee/tea	Plain cookies, 4
		Coffee/tea
Dinner		
Beef roast, 3 ounces	Beef roast, 4 ounces	Beef roast, 5 ounces
Baked potato, 1 medium	Baked potato, 1 medium	Baked potato, 1 medium
Broccoli, ½ cup	Broccoli, ½ cup	Broccoli, ½ cup
Milk, skim, 1 cup	Roll, 1	Roll, 1
	Margarine, 1 teaspoon	Margarine, 2 teaspoons
	Milk, lowfat (1%), 1 cup	Milk, lowfat (2%), 1 cup
	Angel food cake (¹⁄₁₆), with strawberries, ½ cup	Angel food cake (¹⁄₁₂), with strawberries, ½ cup, and ice milk, ⅓ cup
Snacks		
Cucumber slices, 1 small cucumber	Peach, fresh, 1 medium	Peach, fresh, 1 medium
Carrot sticks, 3 or 4 strips (2½ to 3 inches long)		Fruit-flavored yogurt, 1 cup
		Banana, 1 small

Source: *Food,* Home and Garden Bulletin Number 228; United States Department of Agriculture.

Fiber

As you get older, a high-fiber diet becomes increasingly important and can be obtained through the increased consumption of fruits and vegetables. Essentially, **fiber** is the indigestible substance in plant food. A high-fiber diet is especially important for maintaining the efficiency of your intestinal track. If there is not regular bulk in your intestines to make the intestinal muscles work, your intestines become "lazy," and you may find yourself needing to rely more on laxatives. Drinking at least seven glasses of fluid a day also helps in this regard.

Cholesterol

Cholesterol is another substance that needs to be monitored closely as you get older. **Cholesterol** is a fatty alcohol manufactured in the body and is associated with heart disease. The amount of saturated fat you consume strongly correlates with your cholesterol levels. If you consume reduced amounts of saturated fat, you have a much better chance of reducing the cholesterol level in your blood. Saturated fat is found mostly in animal fat—in foods such as steaks and chops—and in animal by-products, such as whipped cream, cheese, and milk. Saturated fat is also fairly high in kidneys, shrimp, and lobsters.

The American Heart Association recommends that you limit your diet to about 300 milligrams of cholesterol a day, which is equivalent to approximately one egg. If your cholesterol level is over 150 milligrams, you should try to reduce your saturated fat intake. The American Heart Association also recommends that you reduce the amount of fat in your diet to about 30 percent of your total daily dietary intake and try to keep the amount of saturated fats to about 10 percent.

Table 9.15 shows the cholesterol content of some foods.

Weight and Fat Reduction Myths

Weight and fat reduction myths that need to be dispelled include cellulite, spot reducing, and saunas and steam baths.

Cellulite and Health Spas

For some time there has been a popular myth that there are two kinds of body fat—regular fat and cellulite—and that cellulite is a sort of lumpy, hard fat that can be broken and burned up only through the vigorous massages provided by massage machines found in health spas. The reality, however, is that cellulite is just another word for fat.

Recently, the American Medical Association evaluated the evidence on cellulite and concluded that cellulite is a hoax. Also, the health spa techniques, such as rolling, vibrating, and thumping the body through passive exercise, are completely ineffective in weight reduction. For the body to lose fat, the muscles have to contract and perform work, and the body has to go into negative caloric balance (the amount of energy burning up calories is greater than the number of calories consumed), which results in stored fat being utilized.

Spot Reducing

Spot reducing (exercising specific areas of the body to reduce stored fat) is widely accepted, even though there is no evidence that it works. Generally, overall exercise, such as jogging, swimming, and bicycling, is the most efficient way to burn

Table 9.15 Cholesterol Content of Some Foods

Food	Serving size	Cholesterol (mg)
Milk		
Skim milk	1 cup	7
Whole milk	1 cup	25
Ice cream	¼ cup	50
Meat		
Beef, lean, cooked	3 oz	110
Chicken, flesh only, cooked	3 oz	90
Egg, whole (50 g)	1	255
Egg white (33 g)	1	0
Egg yolk (17 g)	1	255
Fish fillet, cooked	3 oz	60
Heart, cooked	3 oz	130
Kidney, cooked	3 oz	320
Lamb, lean, cooked	3 oz	110
Liver, cooked	3 oz	260
Lobster, cooked	3 oz	170
Mutton, lean, cooked	3 oz	130
Oysters, raw	3 oz (15)	165
Pork, lean, cooked	3 oz	140
Shrimp, flesh only, cooked	3 oz	105
Veal, lean, cooked	3 oz	180
Caviar	1 oz	85
Cheddar cheese	1 oz	30
Creamed cottage cheese	¼ cup	9
Cream cheese	1 oz	35
Fat		
Butter	1 tsp	12
Margarine, all vegetable	1 tsp	0
Margarine, ⅔ animal fat, ⅓ vegetable fat	1 tsp	3
Lard or other animal fat	1 tsp	5

Source: Reprinted by permission from *Understanding Nutrition* by Eleanor Whitney and Eva May Hamilton. Copyright © 1977 by West Publishing Company. All rights reserved (pp. 537–538).

a large number of calories. If the result of such exercise is a negative caloric balance, there is a reduction of fat in the areas of greatest fat concentration, regardless of which part of the body the exercise focused on.

Another thing to keep in mind is that muscle tissue is much more compact than fat tissue. Therefore, a pound of fat takes up a great deal more room than a pound of muscle. Through aerobic exercise, you can burn up fat and at the same time increase your lean body mass, which reduces inches from your girth.

Saunas and Steam Baths

Saunas and steam baths do not increase your metabolic rate and do not melt off fat, as some claim. They can, however, cause dramatic dehydration from the large water losses that occur because of increased body temperature. Although this rapid water loss may be interpreted by some as a weight loss, this "weight loss" will be regained as soon as normal body fluid levels are restored through drinking and eating.

The increased body temperature that results from saunas and steam baths also can dangerously stress the kidneys, heart, and blood vessels. Middle-aged and older individuals and anyone with heart and circulatory problems should be particularly cautious of saunas and steam baths, especially when such methods are accompanied by wrapping in hot towels.

Eating Disorders

Two eating disorders that are especially prevalent in adolescent females are anorexia nervosa and bulimia.

Anorexia Nervosa

Anorexia Nervosa is a state of emaciation brought on by voluntary starvation. Estimates indicate that possibly one out of every two hundred adolescent girls has this disease. Unless it is recognized in its earliest stages, anorexia nervosa is very difficult to treat since the individual simply refuses to eat. Most cases have a psychological basis and represent a form of malnutrition far more serious than that resulting from a lack of food.

Anorexic adolescent females usually experience cessation of menstruation (amenorrhea) and sometimes a fatal electrolyte imbalance. They deny that they are emaciated in spite of a skeletonlike appearance and usually continue to pursue thinness by refusing to eat and maintaining a hyperactive exercise program. Treatment consists of psychiatric as well as nutritional management.

Characteristics of anorexia nervosa include:

1. Avoidance of food, with a loss of at least 25 percent (and sometimes as much as 50 percent) of pre-illness body weight
2. Onset before twenty-five years of age
3. Distorted attitudes toward food, eating, or weight, including denial of illness, enjoyment of extreme weight loss, and unusual hoarding or handling of food
4. No other medical or psychiatric illness that could account for the weight loss
5. At least two of the following:
   a. Cessation of menstrual periods
   b. Lanugo (fine coat of hair over the body)
   c. Slow heartbeat
   d. Periods of overactivity
   e. Episodes of bulimia

Bulimia

A related phenomenon to anorexia nervosa—known as gorge and purge, or **bulimia**—also is seen among adolescents, especially girls. Individuals with bulimia consume unrealistic quantities of food and then induce vomiting or take laxatives to purge themselves of food. This disease has primarily a psychological origin.

Characteristics of bulimia include:

1. Recurrent episodes of binge eating (rapid consumption of a large amount of food in a short period of time, usually less than two hours)
2. At least three of the following:
   a. Consumption of high-calorie, easily ingested food during a binge
   b. Secrecy during a binge
   c. Termination of a binge because of abdominal pain, sleep, or self-induced vomiting
   d. Repeated attempts to lose weight by severely restrictive diets, self-induced vomiting, or use of laxatives
   e. Frequent weight fluctuations greater than ten pounds due to alternating binges and fasts
3. Awareness that eating pattern is abnormal and fear of not being able to stop eating voluntarily
4. Depressed mood and self-deprecating thoughts following binges

Key Terms

Adenosine Triphosphate (ATP)   An energy-rich chemical compound stored in muscle cells; a source of immediate energy

Anorexia Nervosa   An eating disorder characterized by voluntary starvation and a state of emaciation

Bulimia   An eating disorder characterized by alternating binging and purging

Carbohydrates   Chemical compounds containing carbon, hydrogen, and oxygen; examples are sugars and starches; major sources of energy

Carbohydrate Loading   A method by which the amount of glycogen stored by the skeletal muscles is increased through special diets and exercise

Cholesterol   A fatty alcohol produced by the body and by eating certain foods; elevated levels are associated with an increased risk of heart disease

Fasting   Voluntary withdrawal of food from the body

Fats   Food stuffs containing glycerol and fatty acids

Fiber   The indigestible substance in plant food

Glycogen   The storage form of carbohydrates in the body

Kilocalorie   The amount of energy required to raise one kilogram of water one degree centigrade

Minerals Inorganic compounds, some of which are nutrients vital to body function; examples include phosphorus, calcium, potassium, sodium, iron, and iodine

Obesity Excessive body fat (a male who has over 20 percent body fat and a female who has over 30 percent body fat)

Phosphocreatine A chemical that can donate its phosphate to form ATP in the muscle

Polyunsaturated Fat A fatty acid that lacks four or more hydrogen atoms and has two or more double bonds between carbons

Protein Organic material that regulates body processes and builds and repairs body tissue

Saturated Fat A fatty acid carrying the maximum possible number of hydrogen ions; usually, saturated fats remain solid at room temperature

Vitamins Organic compounds that regulate a number of body processes and that are used in the metabolism of carbohydrates and fats

10

Special Considerations

This chapter deals with a variety of special considerations and problems associated with rigorous physical exercise and is divided into five major areas: (1) common injuries, (2) environmental problems, (3) drugs used to improve athletic performance, (4) maintaining fitness with age, and (5) females and exercise. The section on common injuries deals with injuries to the ligaments, tendons, muscles, and bones and also offers tips on prevention and treatment. The next section concerns exercise and such environmental problems as altitude and warm and cold weather. Special precautions and clothing requirements also are discussed. The section on drugs includes information on steroids, amphetamines, alcohol, and dimethyl sulfoxide (DMSO). How age affects performance and exercise intensity levels is examined in the fourth section. The final section in the chapter deals with females and exercise and includes information on how exercise affects menstruation, pregnancy, and childbirth.

Common Injuries

Many of the injuries that occur during exercise are avoidable. Some athletes are injured because they push themselves too hard and too long, or they take unnecessary risks, such as running, for example, over rough and uneven terrain, where injuries are more likely to occur. Also, many individuals are unaware of how easily they can injure themselves. They launch into such activities as tennis and racquetball, which require a lot of repetitions, without a proper warm-up. As a result, the continuous hitting and running movements required in these sports greatly stress muscles, tendons, and ligaments, causing breakdowns, inflammation, and pain. Even well-conditioned individuals who have played tennis for a long time can be afflicted with an inflamed elbow from overuse. Individuals who do a lot of rope jumping or jogging on hard surfaces run the risk of tendon injuries and stress fractures.

Probably the most common injury to the average exerciser, however, is tendinitis. Tendinitis occurs when the tendon is overstressed during exercise. The resulting inflammation and pain may make the area tender and sore for a long time. A good example is jumper's knee, which is an inflammation of the tendon where it attaches to the patella of the kneecap. Jumper's knee usually is the result of small tears in the tendon that have not healed properly. This condition is most common in basketball players and high jumpers, but also can occur in individuals who do a lot of running, jogging, or jumping.

In any exercise or sport in which you participate, make sure that you (1) warm up properly, (2) don't overstress the muscles and joints at the beginning of an activity, and (3) use moderation in repetitive activity. If you don't, you may find yourself suffering from one or more of the common injuries discussed in the sections that follow.

Sprains and Strains

A **sprain** is an injury to a ligament, a fibrous tissue that holds bones together and stabilizes them to form a joint. A ligament has very little elasticity, and if it is stretched beyond its elastic limit, the result may be a permanent injury. In some cases, the ligament may even rupture and break.

Ligament sprains are very common injuries in sports, occurring frequently in the knees and ankles. Many times, a ligament sprain results in immediate pain, but the degree of pain is not always related to the severity of the injury. Less severe ligament injuries may be very painful, while more severe ligament injuries, particularly around the knee, may become painless in a few minutes. If a ligament is completely torn, there may be an absence of pain but abnormal motion when the joint is moved.

The treatment for a ligament sprain generally involves protecting the ligament until it has the opportunity to grow together. A unique characteristic of the new growth after injury is that it does not consist of more ligament tissue, but rather heals with a scar. Sometimes, surgeons suture the torn ligament together so that the scar that connects the two ends will be shorter. Excessive scar tissue can predispose the joint to further injury.

A **strain** is an injury to a muscle or tendon and results when the muscle or tendon is pulled excessively or torn. A tendon is the end of the muscle that attaches to the bone. A tendon is elastic, but in some cases its elasticity is limited, and the tendon can be overstretched and pulled away from the bone. Often, a strain is accompanied by the swelling and bleeding of soft tissue, and this may increase the severity of the pain. As with a ligament sprain, the degree of pain associated with muscle or tendon strain may not be related to the severity of the injury.

There is some debate as to how a strain should be treated. One method involves actively stretching the muscle and tendon throughout the healing process so that the muscle or tendon does not heal shortened, which could lead to subsequent injuries. Another treatment prohibits all activity until the muscle and tendon heal. Then the muscle is gradually stretched to its normal length.

Bone Growth and Injury

The long bones in the body, before reaching maximum length between the ages of sixteen and eighteen, are divided into three separate parts—two ends and a shaft. The ends are connected to the bone shaft by cartilage (semielastic hard tissue covering bones) at a location called the growth plate. The cells of the growth plate eventually mature and fuse the ends of the bones to the shaft to form one solid bone. An injury to the growth plate can damage these cell layers and prevent them from growing properly. As a result, the bone may be deformed or not grow as long as it should have. It is therefore vital that anytime a child injures a bone or joint in an arm or leg that the injury be carefully examined by a physician to determine if the growth plate has been damaged.

Leg Cramps

Cramps are sustained muscle contractions and usually occur in the calf muscle and the lower leg. Early research indicated that cramps resulted from the salt loss that occurred because of excessive sweating. More recent research, however, indicates that cramps may result from a reduction in fluid volume. Therefore, an individual who has frequent cramps in hot weather should try to drink as much fluid as possible (hydrate) before and during rigorous activity.

When a muscle goes into a cramp, it squeezes against the artery and partially cuts off the flow of blood. A reduced flow of blood to the muscle (ischemia) results in pain. Generally, when the muscle goes into **muscle tetanus** (sustained contraction), the best treatment is to stretch the muscle by extending the joint or to press gradually on the body of the muscle, forcing it to stretch. This allows blood to flow to the muscle again, thereby reducing the spasm and pain.

A muscle that has gone into tetanus or that has been injured should not be vigorously massaged. In these situations, massage actuates the stretch reflex, which increases the muscle spasm and leads to further pain and swelling. Generally, massage should be used for body relaxation. During massage, small skin receptors set off a reflex activity, which relaxes the body. Massage also results in the dilation of blood vessels close to the skin surface, which may aid in the return of blood flow to the limb.

Tennis Elbow

Tennis elbow is pain in the upper arm near the elbow and is caused by injury to the muscles that extend the wrist. This affliction gets its name because of the constant hand and wrist flexing and extension of the forearm during tennis that can lead to injury and produce severe pain. In some cases, tennis elbow can be disabling to the point where the person no longer can shake hands or move the hand in a rotating motion.

Generally, X rays of tennis elbow show no sign of change in the bone. In some cases, there may be swelling and inflammation of the tendon (tendinitis). Aspirin is sometimes effective in reducing the pain, and avoiding tennis for two weeks may be the best remedy. In some cases, cortisone is injected into the area of pain; this results in immediate relief, but the pain, unfortunately, returns in a few hours. In very severe cases, surgery is a possibility since the muscle attachment may have pulled away from the bone.

Shinsplints

Shinsplints is a term given to a number of injuries that produce pain in the lower leg. The symptoms are pain on the inner side of the shinbone (tibia) in the front part of the leg. The pain usually is associated with running or jogging. Sometimes, it comes on very slowly and eventually may become quite severe. In some cases, the muscle may even pull away from the bone, or there may be small tears in the muscle where it attaches to the shinbone. In other cases, the pain may be due to a stress fracture, blocked circulation, lowered arch, or damage to nerves in the leg. The condition generally does not result in permanent disability.

The best cure for shinsplints is rest. Wearing good shoes with a firm heel support and avoiding running on hard surfaces sometimes can prevent or reduce the severity of this kind of injury. Running in a reversed direction on a curved track along with concentrating on a heel-to-toe foot stride also have been found to be preventative measures.

Stress Fractures

Stress fractures are very small, minute cracks appearing in any bone that has been stressed repeatedly in such activities as jogging on hard surfaces or jumping for long periods of time. Although a stress fracture becomes painful and during activity is very tender to the touch, this condition cannot be detected in an X ray until two or three weeks after the injury. For this reason, it is important that you don't ignore the pain and continue with your activity, since then an actual break can occur in the bone.

Achilles Tendon Problems

A common running injury occurs in the Achilles tendon, the tendon that connects your calf muscle with your heel. Under the normal stress of running, small tears may occur in the Achilles tendon, but they normally heal in a short time. Once the tendon has been weakened by small tears, however, stair climbing, running up a hill, or similar activities may cause additional tearing. If the leg is continually stressed by exercise, the tendon may become inflamed.

Treatment for an inflamed Achilles tendon consists of ice massage twice a day. If the tendon is torn, ice massage and a heel lift (a small piece of material placed under the heel in the shoe to slightly elevate the heel), along with a four- to six-week layoff from exercise, are recommended. If the tear requires surgery, it is important to consult an orthopedic expert who knows something about the problems of runners.

Preventing Injuries through Proper Shoe Selection

Jogging or running with improperly fitting or poor-quality shoes can result in a variety of back, knee, ankle, and foot problems. When selecting a shoe, keep some basic principles in mind:

1. Purchase a quality shoe. A number of good brands are on the market. Be wary of so-called low-priced running shoes. Remember—you are going to spend many hours in them in all kinds of conditions. So don't be afraid to invest a few extra dollars.

2. Solicit advice about what shoe to purchase from some of your running friends, and check a few speciality stores.

3. If you run on a grass or dirt surface, you need less cushion in the shoe but good traction and stability. If you run on pavement, you need adequate cushioning. However, be careful because too much cushion leads to reduced stability.

4. Do you have a rigid foot or a floppy foot? If you have a rigid foot, the wear spots will be on the outside of your shoe. You probably should select a cushioned shoe that is slip-lasted. If you have a floppy foot, your shoe will wear in various spots on the sole where your foot pushes against the ground. You need a more stable shoe with a little less cushion and a board last (wider form).

5. Do you have a straight foot or a curved foot? If you have a straight foot and wear a curved shoe, you will feel pressure on the outside of each foot. If you have a curved foot and wear a straight shoe, you will feel pressure on your toes. The shape of your shoe should correspond to the shape of your foot. Be sure there are no areas of pressure or pain or a feeling of binding.

Environmental Problems

Hundreds of thousands of individuals who live in a variety of extreme climatic conditions in the United States actively participate in year-round sports. Yet, few cross-country and downhill skiers, hikers, and mountaineers understand the environmental problems associated with high altitudes and cold; few marathon runners and tennis players understand the environmental problems associated with extremely hot climates. Exercise in cold and hot climates without taking the proper precautions may not only lead to slight discomfort but also to serious injury and death.

Exercise in Hot Weather

Exercise in hot environments increases the need for an excess amount of blood flow to the working muscles and also to the skin to maintain body temperature. If the amount of blood necessary to meet the demands exceeds the amount the heart can pump out, a type of circulatory shock or overload occurs. This overload can result in problems with temperature regulation, accompanied by symptoms of dizziness and fainting. In some cases, there may be serious medical consequences.

To avoid problems when exercising in hot weather, begin with moderate exercise and gradually increase to the desired intensity. This gives the human body time to physiologically acclimate itself to the demands made by high temperatures. For example, the heart rate generally decreases, and the amount of blood that flows through the skin decreases, which allows more blood to flow through the deep muscles, where it is needed for the exercise. Also, blood pressure is more adequately maintained, sweating is more efficient, and the sweat that is produced evaporates more effectively. You also lose less salt. In addition to those physiological changes, you are more resistant to dizziness, fainting, and nausea, which are common problems for individuals who exercise in hot weather.

Also important when exercising in hot weather is the frequent ingestion of water and the wearing of clothing that allows for a large skin surface and sweat evaporation. Wear light, porous, short-sleeved shirts and shorts and avoid long socks and warm-up suits. It also is important to protect the top of your head from overheating. In severe heat, a wet cloth, handkerchief, or sock on the top of your head underneath your hat will prove invaluable in keeping the top of your head cool.

Other hot-weather exercise topics include water substitutes, salt needs in hot weather, water loss from exercise in a hot environment, sweating, and long-distance running under very warm conditions.

Water Substitutes

Water substitutes—or as they are more commonly called, sweat replacers—are used frequently by athletes who exercise in hot weather. Gatoraid is one example.

They are mixtures of glucose, sodium, chloride, potassium, magnesium, calcium, and water—all substances that the body loses through sweat during exercise in intense heat. Sweat replacers put these important substances back into the system more efficiently than simply water. Even though these mixtures resemble the composition of sweat (except for the glucose), they probably are absorbed less rapidly than water because of the glucose, which tends to slow down absorption. In fact, it takes an hour for the stomach to absorb one liter of water; it takes even longer for it to absorb a liter of sweat replacer. A good replenishing drink aside from plain water is a mixture of one part orange juice to four parts water.

Salt Needs in Hot Weather

The normal daily intake of salt is about ten to twelve grams. Even under very severe conditions, you do not lose more than thirteen to seventeen grams of salt a day. The only time you need to take in salt is when you are losing very large quantities of water (four to six quarts of water within a twelve-hour period), which is a very rare condition in athletic events.

Normally, the amount of salt needed can be supplied to the body through a normal diet, and regular use of salt tablets is a questionable practice when conditions are not severe. Also keep in mind that more water than salt is lost during exercise. Therefore, taking salt tablets without an adequate amount of water is far worse than taking no salt tablets at all.

Water Loss

In hot weather, the weight lost from exercising over short periods of time is primarily due to water loss, not a breakdown of fatty tissue. This weight quickly returns when you eat and drink. More important, however, is that a large water loss can be very dangerous.

The best way to determine your water loss is to weigh yourself before and after exercise. Water loss of 3 percent or less of total body weight is fairly safe, 5 percent or less is borderline, but anything over 7 percent can severely affect the functioning of the heart and circulatory system. It is possible to lose six to seventeen pounds of water within twenty-four hours, and this amount of water lost through exercise must be replaced. If it isn't, the body stops producing sweat, body temperature increases sharply, and an imbalance in electrolytes occurs. (Sodium, potassium, and chloride collectively are referred to as **electrolytes**, and they are present in the body in the form of electrically charged particles called ions. Electrolytes' main function is to control fluid exchange in various body tissues.)

It is not uncommon for a person exercising in hot weather to lose considerable amounts of water and not feel thirsty. You should not depend on your natural feeling of thirst to satisfy your body's needs for water replacement.

Sweating

During rigorous exercise, efficient sweating indicates that the body is responding well to the increase in body temperature. Sweating provides water to the surface area of the skin; there the water evaporates into the air, which cools the body and regulates body temperature.

Because the skin surface is important for sweat evaporation, large areas of the skin should be exposed for efficient sweating. Approximately 55 percent of all sweat is lost from the trunk area of the body, 25 percent is lost from the head and the upper limbs, and 25 percent is lost from the lower limbs. When exercising in hot weather, wear light, loose-fitting clothing, such as shorts and a shirt made of light-weight material or a cotton/polyester blend with large holes. Avoid hoods, towels around your head and neck, rubber belts, and sweat suits, which increase body temperature and cause fluid loss.

Long-Distance Running in Hot Weather

Competitive races covering distances over ten miles should not be conducted when the temperature exceeds twenty-eight degrees centigrade or eighty-eight degrees Fahrenheit (wet bulb). During periods of the year when the daylight temperature exceeds these limits, races should be conducted before 9:00 A.M. or after 4:00 P.M. Race sponsors should provide fluids that contain small amounts of sugar (less than 2.5 grams glucose per 100 milliliters of water) and electrolytes, such as sodium and potassium. Frequent ingestion of fluids during competition is important, as is consuming thirteen to seventeen ounces of fluid ten to fifteen minutes before the race. There should be water stations at every 2- to 2.5-mile interval for all races ten miles and longer. Unless these simple precautions are taken, endurance running in hot climates can result in serious physical disability and sometimes death.

Exercise in Cold Weather

Exercise in cold weather is generally less stressful on the circulatory system because there is less body heat production. Running or cycling in cold weather, however, can reduce body temperature because of the chill factor, especially if there is a wind. In these cases and also when the temperature drops below forty degrees Fahrenheit, you need some protection. Make sure that your head and hands are covered. Materials made from wool or polypropylene are excellent. Wind or rain suits made from Goretex or PTFE-film keep you dry and also allow heat to escape. When it is extremely cold, dress in layers, so that when you exercise, you can take off clothing as your body temperature goes up.

It also is important to keep in mind that retention of heat causes excessive sweating, even in freezing weather. If your skin surface is covered by heavy clothing, sweat cannot evaporate efficiently and cool the body. As a result, body temperature rises further, and large amounts of sweat permeate socks and underclothing. When you stop exercising, the sweat-soaked clothing may freeze, which could result in some very severe consequences.

Altitude Sickness

Many individuals experience headaches, feelings of drowsiness, insomnia, and a lack of appetite at altitudes as low as twenty-six hundred meters. This is called **altitude sickness.** In serious cases of altitude sickness, fluid accumulates in the lungs, which sometimes is erroneously diagnosed as pneumonia. If individuals in this condition are given antibiotics without being taken to lower altitudes, they may die. Altitude sickness also produces an intolerance to fatty foods that may result in nausea and vomiting. In some cases, the symptoms of altitude sickness are paradoxically euphoric, rather than disabling, and the individual may experience feelings of well-being, especially during the first night. Most people are affected to some degree by altitude sickness at altitudes over forty-three hundred meters.

The most effective remedy for altitude sickness is gradual descent to lower altitudes to minimize the symptoms. A diet high in carbohydrates and low in fat and the avoidance of strenuous exercise at high altitudes also can reduce the severity of altitude sickness.

Air Pollution and Exercise

In some parts of the United States, the atmosphere contains many pollutants, such as nitrogen oxide, sulfur oxide, carbon dioxide, and particulate matter like dust and solid particles. Also, ozone, which results from the sun's action on nitrogen dioxide, and hydrocarbon from automobile exhaust are major pollutants. Some evidence indicates that ozone can reduce an individual's ability to bring in oxygen and thus interferes with such aerobic activities as long-distance running and jogging. Also, particulate matter and fumes can increase resistance to air flow to the lungs and result in less efficiency. Pollutants not only affect physical performance—their long-term toxic effects on the lungs and circulatory system are well documented.

Drugs Used to Improve Athletic Performance

The use of drugs by amateur and professional athletes to improve performance is currently a topic of public debate. Athletes are always looking for that "extra edge" that will give them the advantage over their opponents. When only a hundredth of a second may separate first place from last, it is little wonder that drugs that claim to improve performance gain acceptance.

Such drugs as anabolic steroids and amphetamines are used in an attempt to increase muscle strength and endurance and delay the onset of fatigue, while in fact, these drugs can adversely affect performance and lead to long-term health problems. Alcohol and cigarettes also can pose a serious threat if used prior to and during physical exercise. Dimethyl sulfoxide (DMSO), while not used to stimulate or improve performance, is being experimentally administered to reduce muscle soreness and thereby allow athletes to continue performing or competing. How exercise affects disease resistance also is discussed in this section.

Anabolic Steroids

Anabolic steroids are basically synthetic hormones that are similar to the male hormone testosterone, which builds body tissue and also has a masculinizing effect on the body. Most research is contradictory with regard to whether taking anabolic steroids can actually produce increased muscle bulk. Any increase in muscle size probably is due to steroids causing fluid to be retained in the muscle. Generally, an increase in muscle size comes only from training.

In addition to their dubious ability to increase muscle bulk, anabolic steroids have some very serious side effects. For example, if anabolic steroids are administered to a male athlete, his testes cease to produce testosterone and depend entirely upon the external source of the hormone. Side effects also can include irritability and other personality changes. In some instances, prolonged use of steroids may cause tumors of the liver and kidney. The administration of steroids before puberty can result in early closure of the epiphysis (the growth plates of the bones), resulting in shortened or retarded growth.

When large doses of anabolic steroids are administered to women for long periods of time, such male characteristics as facial hair and a deeper voice may develop, and the women increase their chances of having liver or kidney tumors.

Amphetamines

Amphetamines are a group of drugs that stimulate the central nervous system of the body. Some side effects are increased heart rate, blood flow, and blood pressure and metabolism. Very little scientific evidence, however, indicates that amphetamines improve performance or increase endurance. Most of the studies, in fact, report that the drugs have very little effect.

One of the dangers of taking amphetamines during exercise is that the individual may not be sensitive to the symptoms of fatigue and exhaustion and may overstress the body, which sometimes irreparably damages the heart.

Alcohol

Alcohol acts as a general depressant on the central nervous system. Problems occur when alcohol is consumed in quantities that exceed the body's capability to metabolize it. Unlike most substances, alcohol is absorbed directly from the stomach. An adult can metabolize about one-half to three-fourths of an ounce of pure alcohol per hour. (Two ounces of a 100-proof bourbon, for example, equals one ounce of pure alcohol.) One ounce of pure alcohol produces a blood alcohol level of 0.5 percent in a large adult. Four ounces of pure alcohol produce a blood alcohol level of 0.20 percent, resulting in severe intoxication. A blood alcohol level over 2.0 percent produces coma and sometimes death.

Alcohol interferes with coordination, vision, and judgment. It also slows reaction time and can produce severe motor disturbances, such as staggering, and impaired sensory perception. Long-term damage to the brain and liver may also result from use of alcohol. In addition, alcohol negatively affects the controlling impulses to the heart. Thus, individuals who exercise after drinking alcohol run the risk of irregular heartbeats. Increased heart rate also is common because of alcohol's depressant effect upon the central nervous system, which is unable to regulate and control the heart properly. Finally, evidence indicates that alcohol taken prior to rigorous physical activity can result in a reduced blood supply to the heart tissue. For all of these reasons, alcohol obviously has no place in physical exercise.

Dimethyl Sulfoxide (DMSO)

Dimethyl sulfoxide (DMSO) is a by-product of wood pulp that has been used as an industrial solvent, as a paint thinner, and also by veterinarians, who use it to treat injuries to large animals. Because DMSO is a solvent, when placed on the skin it can carry anything that is on the skin, such as deodorants, after-shave lotions, soap film, cosmetics, and other contaminants, into the circulatory system. One side effect of DMSO is that it produces a garlicky bad breath.

Recently, athletes have been using DMSO to deal with acute and chronic joint and muscle pain, although evidence is limited as to its exact function in decreasing pain. In some cases with humans, DMSO has rapidly reduced pain, swelling, and disability to muscles and joints. It is generally more effective in acute injuries than in chronic injuries. One of the difficulties of using DMSO is determining on which injuries it has a greater effect. Evidence is limited in this area.

One of the major problems with DMSO is the lack of control over its manufacture, thereby making it impossible to ensure the quality of the drug. Also, by using DMSO, you may be forsaking other significant aids for decreasing the injury—looking for a quick cure or fix rather than accepted therapy, such as ice, rest, stretching, strapping, taping, and so on.

Exercise and Disease Resistance

There is very little evidence to link rigorous exercise with increased susceptibility to disease. It is possible that hormones released by the adrenal glands during stress from overexertion may inhibit certain immune responses, but the facts are not clear as to whether this leads to an increase in the infection process. No evidence at the present time indicates that the physical stress resulting from athletic activity predisposes an individual to susceptibility to infection.

Another related question is whether stress resulting from physical activity can aggravate an already existing infection. Again, there is very little evidence in this regard. If a person has a very high body temperature and an infection, especially a respiratory infection, rigorous physical activity can cause sudden changes in body temperature and can irritate the infected tissue, thereby increasing the infection.

Exercising when you have a virus infection, runny nose, sneezing, aching, and other symptoms of mild upper respiratory infection is not advised. Working off the infection through exercise even may be dangerous since the virus could find its way to your heart muscle, resulting in myocarditis, which inflames and damages the heart muscle. Avoid exercise until your symptoms have disappeared.

One final note about how exercise affects disease resistance is that individuals with asthma who overexert themselves through exercise or breathe in too much cold air may induce bronchial spasms. Also, some evidence indicates that a small percentage of the population who do not have classical asthma can bring on asthmatic-like symptoms by rapidly breathing in cool air. This is a common occurrence among runners in cool environments.

Maintaining Fitness with Age

The health of an individual at each stage of the aging process is based upon the foundations that were layed down in previous years. Because we all age, it is necessary to know what those changes are and how they can be affected by our living habits, such as nutrition and exercise. Only recently has there been interest in what causes the body to prematurely age or run down.

In addition, exercise for the older person is a comparatively recent phenomenon brought about by a change in social mores and a new perception of the role of exercise in life. Today it is not uncommon to see older people jogging, swimming, and engaging in a variety of activities. The increased number of individuals exercising has generated an increased interest in the effects of exercise on the body. The interest in exercise is not only limited to maintaining physical fitness but also involves its relationship with chronic diseases associated with aging, such as heart disease, diabetes, high blood pressure, and osteoporosis.

Statistics on population trends indicate that we are becoming a nation of older people. As a result, there is an increased need for evaluation of the aging process, its effects on physical performance, and the roles of exercise and nutrition in preserving our health and vitality.

Aging and Performance Levels

In general, an individual's ability to perform physical activities declines with age. This area, however, has not been researched thoroughly because a number of factors make it very difficult to assess. For example, as a person ages, he or she is more susceptible to a number of diseases, which can affect physical performance. Also, because of the sedentary nature of most Americans, it is very difficult to find an old population to compare with a young population at equal levels of physical activity. Very few studies have analyzed individuals from birth to old age within the same population.

Research, however, has been able to establish a number of facts about how aging affects our bodies. First, overall muscle strength decreases slightly with age. An individual generally achieves maximum strength at about thirty years of age, and there is a slight decrease from that time on. Even at the age of sixty, however, a person's loss of maximum muscle strength is only about 10 to 20 percent of that at age thirty. Research also has determined that the muscles' ability to increase in size (muscle hypertrophy) decreases with age. Muscle hypertrophy, however, usually is not responsible for an increase in strength level. Strength increases usually are due to better coordination and skill and to nerve innervation. An individual's maximum heart rate (220 minus age) also decreases with age—about forty beats per minute from the age of twenty to the age of seventy-five. Cardiac output, the amount of blood pumped out by the heart, decreases after the age of thirty by approximately 1 percent per year. Also, peripheral blood flow to the extremities decreases. An increased resistance to blood flow caused by hardening of the arteries results in higher blood pressure. Research also has established that the amount of air an individual can bring into the lungs decreases with age because of decreased efficiency of the muscle of the chest wall and also of the lung tissue itself. Two final changes with age: body fat tends to increase as individuals get older, and reaction time slows down.

The physiological trainability of an older individual is roughly equal to that of a young adult when expressed on a relative basis, taking into account the various physiological factors of aging. In other words, older persons exercising in an individualized program can maintain levels of strength, cardiac output, and oxygen uptake that are as reasonable for them as are comparable programs for younger individuals.

Types of Exercise for Older Individuals

An exercise program for an older person should consist of flexibility exercises, calisthenics, and a continuous fast walking or jogging program. Stretching exercises and light calisthenics stimulate the muscles and circulation and also maintain good joint flexibility. In addition, they put a slight load upon the heart. However, it also is important to engage in some continuous, rhythmic activity, such as fast walking or jogging, which is of greater benefit to the cardiovascular system. Heart rate should reach levels of about 112 to 120 beats per minute. The flexibility exercises and calisthenics should be done every day, while the jogging or fast walking exercise is important at least three times a week.

The specific level of fitness needed to mitigate cardiac and other health risk factors in older individuals is an important but still unanswered question. Considerable research indicates that the training level necessary for the heart is approximately 70 percent of maximum. This may not be an appropriate standard, however, for individuals over sixty. It has been found that training responses of the heart in individuals over sixty years of age can be elicited at heart rates as low as 90 to 100 beats per minute. Well-conditioned individuals over sixty years of age require heart rates of approximately 103 to 106 beats per minute to produce a training stimulus. The important point to remember is that training response levels are produced at far lower exercise intensities than was first thought. Older individuals should start at very low heart rate levels—under 100 beats per minute—and increase progressively. The intensity level of the exercise, not the type of exercise, is the critical factor, and the pulse rate should be monitored very carefully. While a younger person usually can proceed rapidly with increasing levels of activity, the older person should take care to gradually increase the exercise load and to recheck with a physician every six weeks early in the program.

Finally, it is important for older individuals to avoid sudden, rigorous bursts of exhaustive anaerobic activity, such as sprinting or weight lifting, and to concentrate mainly on endurance activities that are moderate and rhythmic in nature, such as jogging, walking, swimming, and bicycling.

Aging and the Benefits of Exercise

Considerable evidence indicates that the physiological consequences of aging increase if the cardiovascular and respiratory systems are weak. Regular and rhythmic exercise that increases the heart and respiratory rates, then, is an extremely important factor in maintaining health during the older years.

Older individuals derive a number of benefits from physical conditioning. First, evidence indicates that the process of aging is delayed. Also, the ability of older individuals to transport oxygen increases, which increases their aerobic capacity to do work for longer periods of time. There also is some indication that physical conditioning can decrease blood pressure, improve breathing capacity, and make the muscles of the respiratory system more efficient. Other research shows that degenerative bone changes, such as osteoporosis, can be reduced through exercise, which prevents the bones from losing organic matter. Also, older people who engage in exercise programs benefit from improved joint mobility. In addition, such conditions as chronic lung disease, diabetes, coronary artery disease, and angina pain tend to be less severe in older individuals who are physically fit. Finally, some evidence indicates that arteriosclerosis is reduced in individuals who engage in long-term, continuous exercise. All of this adds up to an increase in life expectancy.

Whatever benefit an older person derives from exercise depends upon the type, intensity, and duration of the exercise the person participates in. For example, an older person who has been jogging three to five days a week at a training effect level for many years can expect greater benefits than an individual who plays a round of golf each week.

Nutrition and Aging

Research also indicates that the physiological consequences of aging increase if a nutritionally sound diet is not maintained. While the energy needs of older people remain fairly constant, the digestive process slows down and the amount of nutrients absorbed is reduced. Therefore, the quality of the diet has added importance. More nutrients need to be derived from less food. The decreased energy requirements are due to a decrease in basal metabolism, which is about 10 percent slower for every ten years over sixty.

Older people should observe the following basic principles of nutrition, whether they are exercising or not:

1. Take in fewer overall calories.
2. Increase slightly the amount of protein in the diet.
3. Reduce the amount of fat in the diet.
4. Ensure that sufficient complex carbohydrates are in the diet.
5. Maintain appropriate vitamin and mineral levels, especially vitamin C, iron, and calcium.
6. Include adequate fiber, fruits, vegetables, and whole grains in the diet.
7. Ingest adequate water (six to seven glasses a day).

Females and Exercise

Female athletic competition and participation in physical activities has increased markedly over the past few years, as antiquated social mores regarding women's involvement in sports and exercise have fallen. Because female participation is relatively recent, research on the effects of exercise on the female is scarce. The sections that follow discuss differences between male and female athletes; how exercise affects menstruation, pregnancy, and childbirth; and the iron and calcium needs of females.

Differences between Male and Female Athletes

A number of physiological differences between females and males can result in differences in physical performance. For example, women have a lower center of gravity, which means that they are not as top-heavy as men. As a result, women have better stability, which gives them an advantage in such sports as the martial arts and balancing activities. In addition, women have approximately 26 percent body fat compared to 15 percent for males. The additional fat gives them better buoyancy in the water. This, combined with their lower center of gravity, enables females to maintain body alignment with less physical effort in the water, which results in more efficient swimming movements. The additional fat also serves as insulation, giving women the advantage of being able to maintain body temperature more efficiently in cold water.

Men, on the other hand, exceed women in maximum oxygen consumption during exercise. This is believed to be due to greater cardiac output, blood volume, and oxygen-carrying capacity of the blood. Also, because men have more lean muscle in relationship to total body weight than women, they have about 30 to 40 percent greater absolute strength. Their overall stores of energy-rich compounds, such as ATP, PC, and glycogen, also are greater.

Women's response to physical training in terms of cardiovascular endurance, muscle metabolism, and strength, however, is similar to that of men.

Rigorous Exercise and Menstruation

While a variety of misconceptions and taboos have had women believe otherwise, no research indicates that exercise causes serious health problems during menstruation. Many women do have pain with menstruation, called **dysmenorrhea,** with the degree of discomfort varying from one individual to another. Normally, however, this discomfort should not prevent women from participating in physical activity. As a matter of fact, evidence indicates that physical activity may in some cases reduce the symptoms of menstrual pain.

Some physicians believe that certain exercises, such as skiing, tennis, gymnastics, and rowing, carry greater incidence of menstrual disorder, and they support reduced competition in these areas when women are menstruating. However, little evidence supports this concept.

Recent evidence has shown that approximately one-third of competitive female long-distance runners between the ages of twelve and forty-five experience **amenorrhea** (cessation of menstruation) or **oligomenorrhea** (irregular menstruation) for brief periods. The incidence is usually related to the number of miles run: the longer the distance, the higher the incidence of irregularity. These problems also are found in some gymnasts, swimmers, and dancers, and typically are more common in women who have not given birth or who began menstruating late. Amenorrhea and oligomenorrhea are believed to result from many factors associated with loss of body weight. Generally, a loss that takes the individual below 17 percent body fat is associated with amenorrhea. There is also speculation that rigorous, endurance-type exercise may result in low-level hormone production by the body, which may be the basis for some menstrual cycle irregularities.

Exercise during Pregnancy

No scientific evidence supports the old theory that pregnant women who exercise rigorously develop tense abdominal muscles, which result in problems during delivery. On the contrary, some evidence indicates that women who are athletic have fewer complications during pregnancy, fewer cesarean deliveries, and, generally, shorter labor. If a pregnant woman has medical problems, disease, or other complications, she should seek advice from her obstetrician before undertaking or continuing an exercise program. Extremely rigorous activities that require prolonged endurance or produce a large oxygen debt also are discouraged since these could result in reduced oxygen in the circulatory system and, obviously, reduced oxygen to the fetus. Rhythmic, moderate activity, however, is well advised and safe for both mother and fetus.

Exercise after Childbirth

Women who have just given birth should start exercising as soon as possible if there were no complications and if they have received medical clearance from their physician. They should start slowly because their red blood cell count may be a little low, resulting in feelings of fatigue and shortness of breath. Gradually, over four to six weeks, they should be able to work up to the exercise routine they maintained before they became pregnant. If, during exercise, they feel themselves getting overly tired, they shouldn't force themselves to complete the exercise. Moderation is the key until their body starts responding and they feel as though they can exercise without undue stress.

Female Iron Needs

The average female needs approximately eighteen milligrams of iron a day. (A pregnant woman, however, needs thirty to sixty milligrams.) Since a balanced diet in other nutrients provides approximately only six milligrams of iron per one thousand calories, it is difficult to acquire adequate amounts of iron in a diet below three thousand calories.

Liver is the best source of iron, with no other food group having such a large concentration. Other fairly good sources, however, include meats, cereals, fruits, and vegetables. Eating meat and vegetables at the same meal enhances the absorption of iron. For the same reason, iron supplements should be taken before meals because high-bulk diets reduce iron absorption.

Exercise requires a great deal of oxygen, which is carried by the red blood cells. Red blood cells are composed of iron. Thus, if you are not getting enough iron, your red blood cell count will be low, and your body won't be getting enough oxygen when you exercise, resulting in excessive fatigue. If you are eating a nutritionally balanced diet and taking iron supplements of eighteen milligrams, however, you should have sufficient energy for exercise.

The use of an intrauterine device (IUD) for contraception carries with it the potential loss of more than normal amounts of menstrual blood each period. Thus, a woman who chooses this method of contraception should be certain that her daily iron intake is sufficient to meet this increased need.

Female Calcium Needs and Osteoporosis

Osteoporosis is a disease in which bone tissue degenerates. It ranks closely behind arthritis as a major chronic disease of older people, especially women. Susceptibility to the disease appears to increase with menopause. It may be that the estrogen decreases that accompany menopause hasten the destruction of bone tissue and also decrease the body's absorption rate of calcium, which is vital for the integrity of the bones.

Women who take in very little calcium in their diet also may be more susceptible to osteoporosis. Before menopause, approximately eight hundred milligrams of calcium a day is sufficient for normal nutrition. After menopause, however, women need between one thousand and fifteen hundred milligrams of calcium to maintain bone tissue. Milk, which is one of the best sources of calcium, contains only about one thousand milligrams of calcium per quart. Obviously, then, many older women need calcium supplements to their diets.

Lack of exercise also seems to be a contributing factor to osteoporosis. Exercise helps to stimulate the production of new bone tissue. Also, the activity of muscles working against gravity is crucial in maintaining strong bones. Exercise such as walking and jogging adequately satisfies this need. Even though there is no hard evidence that regular exercise prevents osteoporosis, there is plenty of evidence that shows a lack of physical activity hastens bone loss.

Key Terms

Altitude Sickness   A serious disease encountered at levels as low as twenty-six hundred meters that may produce headaches, insomnia, drowsiness, lack of appetite, nausea and vomiting, and lung congestion

Amenorrhea   An abnormal cessation of menstruation

Amphetamines   A group of drugs that stimulate the central nervous system

Anabolic Steroids   Synthetic hormones that are similar to the male hormone testosterone

Dimethyl Sulfoxide (DMSO)   An industrial solvent that is sometimes used for muscle soreness

Dysmenorrhea   Painful menstruation

Electrolytes   Electrically charged particles, such as sodium, potassium, and chloride

Muscle Tetanus   Sustained muscle contraction

Oligomenorrhea   Irregular menstruation

Osteoporosis   A disease in which the bone tissue degenerates

Shinsplints   A number of injuries that produce pain in the anterior portion of the lower leg

Sprain   An injury to a ligament

Strain   An injury to a muscle or tendon

Stress Fracture   Small, minute cracks in the bone

Tennis Elbow   Pain in the upper arm near the elbow; caused by injury to the muscles that extend the wrist

Coronary Heart Disease and Exercise

Coronary Heart Disease

A major cause of premature death for men and women in the United States is **coronary heart disease,** a disease of the arteries that supply blood to the heart muscle. Coronary heart disease affects over five million people and accounts for over 1.5 million heart attacks each year. It is sometimes referred to as the "silent" disease since some individuals may have no symptoms that indicate its presence. Other individuals, however, may experience such manifestations of the disease as crushing pain in the chest, weakness, breathlessness, or sensations of burning or pressure.

The most common type of coronary heart disease is **atherosclerosis.** Atherosclerosis is caused by an accumulation of plaque on the inner walls of the arteries. **Plaque** forms from deposits of cholesterol, lipids, blood cells, calcium, and tissue debris. Because the coronary arteries are responsible for supplying the heart muscle with oxygen, any interruption in the flow of blood through these vessels can have serious consequences. Plaque can cause artery walls to lose their elasticity. Plaque also may narrow the lining of the artery walls, thus increasing pressure against the walls. If plaque narrows the lining enough, it may completely block the flow of blood. The result is death to tissue that depends on the artery to supply it with nutrients and oxygen.

The reasons for plaque formation are still not well understood. There seems to be agreement, however, that the smooth muscle cells lining artery walls are in some way injured, thus leaving a vulnerable spot for cholesterol and other substances that form plaque to collect.

The heart derives nutrition and oxygen not from the blood that fills its chambers, but from the arteries that lie on its surface. A heart attack, or **myocardial infarction (MI),** occurs when the circulation of blood to the heart muscle is cut

Table 11.1 Coronary heart disease risk factors

Hereditary factors	Internal factors	Habits and environmental factors	Functional factors
Age	Hyperlipemia	Cigarette smoking	Poor cardiovascular fitness
Sex	1. Cholesterol	Diet	
Race	2. Triglycerides	1. Saturated fats	Abnormal electrocardiogram
Family history of premature heart disease	Abnormal lipoprotein distribution	2. Refined sugar	1. At rest
	1. Low density	3. Low-fiber content	2. During exercise
	2. High density	4. Salt	3. After exercise
Hypertension	Hypertension	5. Coffee	Abnormal blood pressure response to exercise
Diabetes	Hyperglycemia	6. Alcohol	
		7. "Soft" water	
Gout	Hyperuricemia	Physical inactivity	1. Hypertension
Hyperlipemia	Hypercoagulability	Obesity	2. Hypotension
Hyperlipoproteinemia		Personality type A	Low vital capacity and related pulmonary flow rates
		Emotional stress	
		Occupation	
		Environmental pollution	

Source: The Possible Place of Stress Testing and Physical Activity to Prevent Coronary Heart Disease. (Coronary heart disease risk factors table), Haskell, W. H., and S. M. Fox. A paper presented at the 59th Annual Meeting of the Southern Medical Association, 1965.

off, resulting in the death of muscle cells in the heart. Atherosclerosis is the most common contributor to heart attacks, but they also can be caused by spasms of the coronary arteries, congenital defects, rheumatic heart disease, and a number of other factors. When the heart tissue dies as a result of arterial blockage, the damaged muscle cells secrete enzymes, which pass into the blood supply. The type and amount of enzymes are one means of diagnosing a heart attack.

Risk Factors of Coronary Heart Disease

As table 11.1 indicates, coronary heart disease is caused by a number of factors. The major factors that have been identified are high blood pressure, high blood cholesterol levels, cigarette smoking, diabetes mellitus, and obesity, and we look at each of these in more detail in the sections that follow. Other factors that appear to play a role in the disease are lack of exercise, certain personality traits, high levels of **triglycerides** (the stored form of free fatty acids) in the blood, and a family history of heart disease. The disease is more common in men than women, and susceptibility increases with age. Many of the risk factors, such as high blood cholesterol and triglyceride levels, high blood pressure, obesity, and smoking, can be controlled and in some cases altered. To determine your risk factor of developing coronary heart disease, take the quiz in table 11.2.

Table 11.2 Assessing your risk factor of developing coronary heart disease

Men

Find the column for your age group. Everyone starts with a score of 10 points. Work down the page adding points to your score or subtracting points from your score.

			54 or younger	55 or older
1. Weight Locate your weight category in the table below. If you are in...			Starting score [10]	Starting score [10]
		weight category A	Subtract 2	Subtract 2
		weight category B	Subtract 1	Add 0
		weight category C	Add 1	Add 1
		weight category D	Add 2	Add 3
			Equals [ ]	Equals [ ]

2. Systolic blood pressure
Use the "first" or "higher" number from your most recent blood pressure measurement. If you do not know your blood pressure, estimate it by using the letter for your weight category. If your blood pressure is...

			54 or younger	55 or older
A	119 or less		Subtract 1	Subtract 5
B	between 120 and 139		Add 0	Subtract 2
C	between 140 and 159		Add 0	Add 1
D	160 or greater		Add 1	Add 4
			Equals [ ]	Equals [ ]

3. Blood cholesterol level
Use the number from your most recent blood cholesterol test. If you do not know your blood cholesterol, estimate it by using the letter for your weight category. If your blood cholesterol is...

			54 or younger	55 or older
A	199 or less		Subtract 2	Subtract 1
B	between 200 and 224		Subtract 1	Subtract 1
C	between 225 and 249		Add 0	Add 0
D	250 or higher		Add 1	Add 0
			Equals [ ]	Equals [ ]

4. Cigarette smoking
If you...
(If you smoke a pipe, but not cigarettes, use the same score adjustment as those cigarette smokers who smoke less than a pack a day.)

		54 or younger	55 or older
do not smoke		Subtract 1	Subtract 2
smoke less than a pack a day		Add 0	Subtract 1
smoke a pack a day		Add 1	Add 0
smoke more than a pack a day		Add 2	Add 3
		Final score [ ]	Final score [ ]

Weight table for men
Look for your height (without shoes) in the far left column and then read across to find the category into which your weight (in indoor clothing) would fall.

Your height ft in	Weight category (lbs) A	B	C	D	
5 1	up to 123	124-148	149-173	174 plus	Because both
5 2	up to 126	127-152	153-178	179 plus	blood pressure
5 3	up to 129	130-156	157-182	183 plus	and blood choles-
5 4	up to 132	133-160	161-186	187 plus	terol are related to
5 5	up to 135	136-163	164-190	191 plus	weight, an esti-
5 6	up to 139	140-168	169-196	197 plus	mate of these risk
5 7	up to 144	145-174	175-203	204 plus	factors for each
5 8	up to 148	149-179	180-209	210 plus	weight category is
5 9	up to 152	153-184	185-214	215 plus	printed at the bot-
5 10	up to 157	158-190	191-220	222 plus	tom of the table.
5 11	up to 161	162-194	195-227	228 plus	
6 0	up to 165	166-199	200-232	233 plus	
6 1	up to 170	171-205	206-239	240 plus	
6 2	up to 175	176-211	212-246	247 plus	
6 3	up to 180	181-217	218-253	254 plus	
6 4	up to 185	186-223	224-260	261 plus	
6 5	up to 190	191-229	230-267	268 plus	
6 6	up to 195	196-235	236-274	275 plus	
Estimate of systolic blood pressure	119 or less	120 to 139	140 to 159	160 or more	
Estimate of blood cholesterol	199 or less	200 to 224	225 to 249	250 or more	

© 1981 American Heart Association

Table 11.2 *Continued*

Women

Find the column for your age group. Everyone starts with a score of 10 points. Work down the page adding points to your score or subtracting points from your score.

		54 or younger	55 or older
1. Weight Locate your weight category in the table below. If you are in...		Starting score [10]	Starting score [10]
	weight category A	Subtract 2	Subtract 2
	weight category B	Subtract 1	Subtract 1
	weight category C	Add 1	Add 0
	weight category D	Add 2	Add 1
2. Systolic blood pressure Use the "first" or "higher" number from your most recent blood pressure measurement. If you do not know your blood pressure, estimate it by using the letter for your weight category. If your blood pressure is...		Equals [ ]	Equals [ ]
	A 119 or less	Subtract 2	Subtract 3
	B between 120 and 139	Subtract 1	Add 0
	C between 140 and 159	Add 0	Add 3
	D 160 or greater	Add 1	Add 6
3. Blood cholesterol level Use the number from your most recent blood cholesterol test. If you do not know your blood cholesterol, estimate it by using the letter for your weight category. If your blood cholesterol is...		Equals [ ]	Equals [ ]
	A 199 or less	Subtract 1	Subtract 3
	B between 200 and 224	Add 0	Subtract 1
	C between 225 and 249	Add 0	Add 1
	D 250 or higher	Add 1	Add 3
4. Cigarette smoking If you...		Equals [ ]	Equals [ ]
	do not smoke	Subtract 1	Subtract 2
	smoke less than a pack a day	Add 0	Subtract 1
	smoke a pack a day	Add 1	Add 1
	smoke more than a pack a day	Add 2	Add 4
5. Estrogen use Birth control pills and hormone drugs contain estrogen. A few examples are *Premarin *Ogan *Menstranol *Provera *Evex *Menest *Estinyl *Meurium		Equals [ ]	Equals [ ]
*Have you ever taken estrogen for five or more years in a row? *Are you age 35 years or older and now taking estrogen?	No to both questions	Add 0	Add 0
	Yes to one or both questions	Add 1	Add 3
		Final score [ ]	Final score [ ]

Weight table for women	Your height ft in	Weight category (lbs)			
		A	B	C	D
Look for your height (without shoes) in the far left column and then read across to find the category into which your weight (in indoor clothing) would fall.	4 8	up to 101	102-122	123-143	144 plus
	4 9	up to 103	104-125	126-146	147 plus
	4 10	up to 106	107-128	129-150	151 plus
	4 11	up to 109	110-132	133-154	155 plus
	5 0	up to 112	113-136	137-158	159 plus
	5 1	up to 115	116-139	140-162	163 plus
	5 2	up to 119	120-144	145-168	169 plus
	5 3	up to 122	123-148	149-172	173 plus
	5 4	up to 127	128-154	155-179	180 plus
	5 5	up to 131	132-158	159-185	186 plus
	5 6	up to 135	136-163	164-190	191 plus
	5 7	up to 139	140-168	169-196	197 plus
	5 8	up to 143	144-173	174-202	203 plus
	5 9	up to 147	148-178	179-207	208 plus
	5 10	up to 151	152-182	183-213	214 plus
	5 11	up to 155	156-187	188-218	219 plus
	6 0	up to 159	160-191	192-224	225 plus
	6 1	up to 163	164-196	197-229	230 plus
Estimate of systolic blood pressure		119 or less	120 to 139	140 to 159	160 or more
Estimate of blood cholesterol		199 or less	200 to 224	225 to 249	250 or more

Because both blood pressure and blood cholesterol are related to weight, an estimate of these risk factors for each weight category is printed at the bottom of the table.

© 1981 American Heart Association

What your score means

0-4	You have one of the lowest risks of heart disease for your age and sex.
5-9	You have a low to moderate risk of heart disease for your age and sex, but there is some room for improvement.
10-14	You have a moderate to high risk of heart disease for your age and sex, with considerable room for improvement on some factors.
15-19	You have a high risk of developing heart disease for your age and sex, with a great deal of room for improvement on all factors.
20 & over	You have a very high risk of developing heart disease for your age and sex and should take immediate action on all risk factors.

Warning

- If you have diabetes, gout, or a family history of heart disease, your actual risk will be greater than indicated by this appraisal.
- If you do not know your current blood pressure or blood cholesterol level, you should visit your physician or health center to have them measured. Then figure your score again for a more accurate determination of your risk.
- If you are overweight, have high blood pressure or high blood cholesterol, or smoke cigarettes, your long-term risk of heart disease is increased even if your risk in the next several years is low.

How to reduce your risk

- Try to quit smoking permanently. There are many programs available.
- Have your blood pressure checked regularly, preferably every twelve months after age 40. If your blood pressure is high, see your physician. Remember, blood pressure medicine is only effective if taken regularly.
- Consider your daily exercise (or lack of it). A half hour of brisk walking, swimming, or other enjoyable activity should not be difficult to fit into your day.
- Give some serious thought to your diet. If you are overweight or eat a lot of foods high in saturated fat or cholesterol (whole milk, cheese, eggs, butter, fatty foods, fried foods), then changes should be made in your diet. Look for the American Heart Association Cookbook at your local bookstore.
- Visit or write your local Heart Association for further information and copies of free pamphlets on many related subjects including
  - Reducing your risk of heart attack
  - Controlling high blood pressure
  - Eating to keep your heart healthy
  - How to stop smoking
  - Exercising for good health

Some words of caution

- If you have diabetes, gout, or a family history of heart disease, your real risk of developing heart disease will be greater than indicated by your score. If your score is high and you have one or more of these additional problems, you should give particular attention to reducing your risk.
- If you are a woman under 45 years or a man under 35 years of age, your score represents an upper limit on your real risk of developing heart disease. In this case, your real risk is probably lower than indicated by your score.
- If you are a woman whose use of estrogen has contributed to a high score, you may want to consult your physician. Do not automatically discontinue your prescription.
- Using your weight category to estimate your systolic blood pressure or your blood cholesterol level makes your score less accurate.
- Your score will tend to overestimate your risk if your actual values on these two important factors are average for someone of your height and weight.
- Your score will underestimate your risk if your actual blood pressure or cholesterol level is above average for someone of your height or weight.

High Blood Pressure

High blood pressure, or **hypertension,** is believed to affect approximately sixty million Americans. It is broadly defined as chronically elevated blood pressure above the normal level considered healthy for your age and sex. **Systolic blood pressure** is the highest level of pressure exerted against the walls of the arteries from ventricular contraction. **Diastolic blood pressure** is the lowest level of pressure exerted against the walls of the arteries during ventricular relaxation. Systolic blood pressure of 140 to 160 millimeters of mercury (mmHg) or diastolic blood pressure of 90 to 95 mmHg is considered borderline hypertension. Systolic blood pressure of 161 mmHg or greater or diastolic blood pressure of 96 mmHg or greater is diagnosed as absolute hypertension. The higher the blood pressure, the greater the incidence of coronary heart disease.

Hypertension may result from kidney disease or a hormonal imbalance. However, 95 percent of the time, the cause is unknown. Increased blood pressure may result when arteries are narrowed or when the volume of blood that moves through the arteries increases. Most researchers believe that the kidneys are involved in the narrowing of the arteries because the kidneys play a role in the release of renin, aldosterone, and norepinephrine, which control arterial wall constriction.

Narrowed arteries tend to resist the flow of blood as it leaves the heart, which places additional pressure on the left ventricle to pump the blood out. If resistance to the flow of blood from the left ventricle continues, the muscle of the ventricle wall enlarges and forms abnormal tissue, which eventually can lead to heart failure. Increased pressure can also lead to stroke and kidney damage.

High blood pressure over a long period of time also results in increased wear and tear on the arteries. Thus, there is always the danger that a weakness in one of the artery walls might rupture, resulting in heart failure, cerebral hemorrhage, or kidney failure.

Many individuals with hypertension may be completely unaware of it. Even mild hypertension (diastolic pressure of 90 to 104 mmHg) may be dangerous. Fortunately, control of hypertension has been aided recently by a number of effective drugs.

Considerable evidence indicates that continuous, rigorous exercise can reduce resting diastolic and systolic blood pressures in middle-aged people. The reduction, however, is most significant in men and women who are leading sedentary lives, who are in poor physical fitness, and who have high blood pressure. Individuals under thirty years of age probably will see no reduction in blood pressure resulting from exercise.

Individuals with high blood pressure should avoid isometric exercises. The sustained muscle contraction required in isometrics causes occlusion of the blood and results in increased pressure in the arteries and the heart. Increases as high as diastolic 20 mmHg during exercise can be very dangerous. In general, people with high blood pressure should avoid lifting and arm-support types of exercises or exercises where the breath is held during lifting.

High Blood Cholesterol Levels

While the complex process that produces atherosclerosis is still not well understood, it *is* known that cholesterol is an important component of arterial plaque. **Cholesterol** is a fatty alcohol produced by the body and by eating certain foods, and it is found in all body cells that serve as building blocks for cell components and hormones. Its exact role in plaque formation is not really clear.

Cholesterol is transported in the blood with three special kinds of proteins, called lipoproteins, which are differentiated by their density: **high-density lipoprotein (HDL), low-density lipoprotein (LDL),** and very low density lipoprotein (VLDL). High-density lipoproteins appear to protect against coronary atherosclerosis, while lower-density lipoproteins seem to promote the disease process. Yet, paradoxically, both HDL and LDL contain cholesterol. It is theorized that HDL works against the atherosclerosis process by resisting the movement of low-density cholesterol into the arterial wall and/or by promoting the influx of cholesterol from the tissues to the liver, where it is broken down and excreted.

The relative distribution of cholesterol into the three types of lipoproteins may be as important as the overall cholesterol level in the blood. Studies indicate that women, lean people, nonsmokers, moderate drinkers, and people who exercise have relatively higher levels of HDL than men, obese people, smokers, nondrinkers, and sedentary people. As yet, the effect of diet on HDL is not clear. It is clear, however, that people vary widely not only in their coronary risk factor but also in their blood composition and their response to diet.

The ratio of total cholesterol to HDL cholesterol should be less than 5 to 1; that is, at least 20 to 25 percent of total cholesterol in the blood should be HDL. The American Heart Association advises that an individual stay below the limit of approximately 300 milligrams of cholesterol a day, or slightly more than the amount found in one egg. On the average, Americans currently consume approximately 450 milligrams daily, with women consuming roughly 350 milligrams and men consuming 550 milligrams.

A promising new method of lowering cholesterol levels involves replacing ordinary oils and margarine in the diet with oils and margarine made of an artificial fat. **Sucrose polyester (SPE),** a compound composed of fatty acids linked with sucrose, cannot be absorbed by the body. Cholesterol eaten in a meal together with SPE is carried out of the body in the feces. More importantly, the cholesterol that the body manufactures also is carried out of the body, lowering total body cholesterol. More research, however, still has to be conducted on this substance.

Smoking

The American Heart Association states that a person who smokes more than one pack of cigarettes a day runs nearly twice the risk of heart attack than a non-smoker. Cigarette smoking both increases the smoker's airway resistance and decreases the amount of oxygen carried in the blood.

Airway resistance is specifically the result of long-term smoking and is caused by narrowing of the bronchial tubes from smoke particles, tar, and constriction of small blood vessels. If severe enough, airway resistance can lead to decreased endurance since there is reduced oxygen exchange, which ultimately results in a reduced oxygen supply to the heart and muscles.

A reduction in the amount of oxygen carried in the blood also is produced by carbon monoxide—the by-product of cigarette smoking. Carbon monoxide has a greater capacity for combining with hemoglobin (the major component of red blood cells, which carry oxygen) than does oxygen. Therefore, when both carbon monoxide and oxygen are present, carbon monoxide is quicker to combine with hemoglobin. And since oxygen and carbon monoxide cannot be carried simultaneously by hemoglobin, the oxygen-carrying capacity of the blood is sharply reduced.

In addition, the nicotine found in cigarettes causes vasoconstriction of the blood vessels, reducing their surface area and the amount of oxygen that can be absorbed into the blood during respiration.

A reduced amount or abnormally low level of oxygen in the coronary circulation results in reduced oxygen to the heart muscle, which can produce ischemia or possible tissue damage. Smoking also results in narrowing or constriction of coronary arteries, further reducing oxygen supply.

Diabetes Mellitus

Diabetes mellitus is a metabolic disorder of energy metabolism caused by an absolute or relative deficiency of insulin. The major problem of diabetes is that glucose has difficulty getting to the cells of the body. Instead, it remains in the blood and builds up to high levels.

Atherosclerosis tends to develop easily in some diabetics, and the arteries become blocked by the formation of plaque. The diseased arteries not only affect the heart but also the eyes and kidneys.

During rigorous exercise, certain diabetics may need more food since exercise has an insulin-like effect. General guidelines are that no extra food is needed for exercise of short duration and modest intensity. During moderate exercise (for example, playing golf), ten to fifteen grams of carbohydrates are allowed per hour. During vigorous exercise (for example, playing basketball and jogging), twenty to thirty grams of carbohydrates may be needed.

Recent evidence indicates that regular exercise can reduce the amounts of sugars and fats in the blood of diabetics.

Obesity

Obesity (excessive body fat) ironically is one of the most important and least understood areas in the science of nutrition. Recently, however, considerable evidence has linked obesity to coronary heart disease. Hypertension occurs about three times as often in obese individuals. Among adults ages twenty through forty-four, overweight individuals are five to six times more likely than others to have hypertension. Also, high blood cholesterol levels occur more than twice as often in the obese as in the nonobese, and the prevalence of diabetes is nearly three times as high. Fat people also die younger from a host of problems, including strokes, heart attacks, and diabetes. In fact, gaining weight appears to precipitate diabetes. Being overweight can cause blood sugar, blood pressure, and blood lipids to climb upward. Fortunately, obesity is reversible in many cases, and if corrected in time, the risk factors also may be reversed.

Physical Activity and Coronary Heart Disease

Regular physical activity has been found to be an essential ingredient in reducing the risk of coronary heart disease. Regular exercise may:

1. Reduce triglyceride levels and increase the levels of high-density lipoproteins that seem to afford some protection against heart disease
2. Affect the pituitary gland, which may, in turn, lower lipid (fat) levels in the blood
3. Result in weight loss, which is a major factor in heart disease
4. Reduce emotional tension, which may increase the body threshold to stress response
5. Result in the regression of atheroma (the blocked portion of the artery) in major arteries

Endurance training may improve metabolic capacity and have a modifying effect on a number of other factors involved in the development of heart disease. Changes in metabolic function, such as decreased resting heart rate, increased myocardial efficiency, peripheral blood distribution, and arterial blood pressure, may all lessen the load on the heart.

The American Heart Association states that, "Exercise training can increase cardiovascular function capacity and decrease myocardial oxygen demand for any given level of physical activity in normal persons as well as most cardiac patients. Regular physical activity is required to maintain the training effects. The potential risk of vigorous physical activity can be reduced by appropriate medical clearance, education, and guidance. Exercise may aid efforts to control cigarette smoking, hypertension, lipid abnormalities, diabetes, obesity, and emotional stress. Evidence suggests that regular, moderate, or vigorous occupational

Table 11.3 Mechanics by which physical activity can reduce occurrence or severity of coronary heart disease

Physical activity increases:	Physical activity decreases:
Coronary collateral vascularization (?)	Serum lipid levels:
Vessel size	Triglycerides
	LDL cholesterol
HDL cholesterol	Glucose intolerance
Myocardial efficiency	Obesity-adiposity
Efficiency of peripheral blood distribution and return	Platelet stickiness
Electron-transport capacity	Arterial blood pressure
Fibrinolytic capability	Heart rate
Red blood cell mass and blood volume	Vulnerability to dysrhythmias
Thyroid function	Neurohormonal overreaction
Tolerance to stress	"Strain" associated with psychic "stress"
Prudent living habits	The size of atheroma
"Joie de vivre"	Collagen accumulation in coronary arteries
Width of coronary artery lumina	
Metabolic turnover of collagen in the heart	

Source: From Fox, S. M., J. P. Naughton, and W. L. Haskell, "Physical Activity and the Prevention of Coronary Heart Disease," in *Annals of Clinical Research* 3:404–432, 1971, Helsinki, Finland.

or leisure time physical activity may protect against coronary heart disease and may improve the likelihood of survival from a heart attack."[*]

There is evidence that much of the improved functional capacity due to exercise is not directly related to the heart. Many times, the improvement in fitness is due to increases in the ability of skeletal muscle cells to extract oxygen more efficiently from the blood. Of course, this phenomenon is also true for heart muscle cells.

Table 11.3 shows the mechanics by which physical activity can reduce the occurrence or severity of coronary heart disease.

Coronary Heart Disease and Stress

Emotional stress may chronically overstimulate a part of the nervous system that can cause spasms in the coronary arteries and produce clumping of the blood platelets (blood cells essential for the clotting of blood). The net effect is a sudden reduction of blood flow to the heart, precipitating irregular beats and a possible heart attack. This condition may result even when there is no severe blockage in the coronary arteries.

[*]American Heart Association, "Subcommittee on Exercise/Cardiac Rehabilitation: Statement on Exercise," *Circulation* 64 (1981):1302–04.

Personality factors appear to play a part in catalyzing this problem. Two personality types have been identified: "hot reactors" and "cold reactors." Hot reactors tend to overrespond physiologically under stress, even though they appear calm on the outside. They may suffer increased blood pressure, coronary artery spasms, and increased resistance to blood flow. Cold reactors, on the other hand, have a normal cardiovascular response to stress, with blood pressure, heart output, and blood vessels changing slowly or only slightly, appropriate to demand. Some evidence indicates that, because a hot reactor's response may be the result of learned experience, the possibly dangerous physiological response may be unlearned through appropriate stress-reduction methods.

Abnormal Heart Size

Recent research has found that a number of young athletes supposedly in excellent physical condition who died suddenly during rigorous physical activity were, in fact, suffering from a disease of the heart muscle known as asymmetrical septal hypertrophy or **idiopathic hypertrophic subaortic stenosis (IHSS)**. The disease is believed to be genetically linked. With this disease, the muscle wall (septum) between the two ventricles of the heart enlarges asymmetrically. This enlargement may block the flow of blood out of the heart. Or the increased abnormal thickness of the muscle may require more oxygen for proper functioning than the normal-sized heart, which means that, during high heart rate levels, the muscle probably would be starved of oxygen and thus malfunction. Individuals who suffer dizziness, light-headedness, blurred vision, fainting, shortness of breath, and heart palpitation, and who also have a history of sudden death in the family would be advised to undergo an echocardiogram and other necessary tests before attempting or continuing rigorous physical activity.

Coronary Rehabilitation

Exercise therapy is a relatively new intervention in the treatment of individuals who have suffered a heart attack or who are prone to coronary heart disease. Recent evidence shows that post-heart-attack individuals involved in exercise rehabilitation programs evidence reduced anxiety and depression, improved self-concept, reduced S.T. depression (which indicates ventricular recovery), reduced blood pressure, reduced resting heart rate, improved exercise capacity, reduced cholesterol and triglyceride levels, and an elevated level of high-density lipoprotein cholesterol.

The primary goal of cardiac rehabilitation is to help patients to reach their optimum physiological and psychological condition. Physical activity should be part of a comprehensive program that includes proper diet, weight control, cessation of smoking, and other social and emotional factors.

While heart attack victims are in the hospital, they should have graded physical activity so that when they leave the hospital, they are able to meet the demands of normal activity, for example, dressing, showering, or walking up a flight of stairs. After leaving the hospital, they should participate in outpatient supervised exercise usually three days a week, while being closely monitored by a physician. Recent evidence indicates that some active physical training can begin as early as three weeks after a heart attack if the exercise is preceded by an intensive physical examination.

The heart attack victim's exercise prescription should be based on careful evaluation with treadmill testing to determine safe parameters, and it should be evaluated periodically. Each individual should maintain a daily training record of intensity, duration, and frequency of exercise. Such activities as walking, jogging, cycling, and swimming are appropriate. Exercising in groups, close, professional supervision, careful evaluation of distress signals, slow warm-ups with gradual increases in the exercise intervals, and periodic heart rate and electrocardiograph monitoring are essential. Cardiac patients involved in any heavy exercise should take some precautions and avoid unnecessary risks.

Fear of exercise is a common problem among those who have suffered a heart attack. Renewed physical exercise, accompanied by physical stress symptoms, may be viewed as dangerous and cause unnecessary anxiety. The anxiety usually decreases, however, as the individual gains confidence through a responsible exercise program.

Key Terms

Atherosclerosis   The most common type of coronary heart disease; caused by the collection of plaque on the inner walls of the arteries

Cholesterol   A fatty alcohol produced by the body and by eating certain foods; elevated levels are associated with an increased risk of heart disease

Coronary Heart Disease   A disease of the arteries that supply blood to the heart muscle

Diabetes Mellitus   A metabolic disorder of energy metabolism caused by an absolute or relative deficiency of insulin

Diastolic Blood Pressure   The lowest level of pressure exerted against the walls of the arteries during ventricular relaxation

High-Density Lipoprotein (HDL)   A class of lipoprotein, high levels of which are thought to provide some protection against coronary heart disease

Hypertension   High blood pressure; chronically elevated blood pressure above the normal level considered healthy for an individual's age and sex

Idiopathic Hypertrophic Subaortic Stenosis (IHSS)   A disease in which the muscle wall (septum) between the two ventricles of the heart enlarges asymmetrically; believed to be genetically linked

Low-Density Lipoprotein (LDL)   A class of lipoprotein, high levels of which are associated with greater risk of coronary heart disease

Myocardial Infarction (MI) Death of muscle cells in the heart because of reduced oxygen supply; heart attack

Obesity Excessive body fat

Plaque Deposits of cholesterol, lipids, blood cells, calcium, and tissue debris, on the inner walls of arteries; a primary factor in atherosclerosis

Sucrose Polyester (SPE) A compound composed of fatty acids linked with sucrose; believed to be a possible aid in reducing blood cholesterol levels

Systolic Blood Pressure The highest level of pressure exerted against the walls of the arteries from ventricular contraction

Triglycerides Stored form of free fatty acids

Exercise and Stress Reduction

The Stress Response

When you experience stress, which can be loosely defined as anything that you experience as a threat to your stability or equilibrium, a portion of your nervous system comes into play to ready the body to meet the demands brought on by this emotional upset. Your heart rate speeds up, your breathing is faster, your pupils dilate, and your muscles become more tense, resulting in an overall heightened mental and physical awareness. This phenomenon is referred to as the **stress response.**

Whether you suffer from stress or thrive on it, your system must be prepared to withstand it. The stress response readies your body to deal with threats efficiently and effectively. It gives your body the stimulus to perform amazing feats, both mental and physical; yet, at the same time, it also can wreak havoc on your health. If the stress is prolonged, it can weaken your body defenses, accelerate the aging process, and lead to chronic disease.

Table 12.1 shows important life events and the degree of stress associated with each measured on a point scale.

Generally, the stress response can be broken down into the three stages defined by Hans Seyle: (1) the alarm reaction stage, (2) the resistance stage, and (3) the exhaustion stage.

The **alarm reaction stage,** or fight or flight response, is the initial reaction of your body to stress. This response mobilizes the body's resources for immediate physical activity. Increased activity of the sympathetic nervous system and su-

Table 12.1 Events people perceive as stressful

People ranked these events, according to how stressful they perceived them to be, on a scale from 1 to 100. Note that some "happy" events are included here. Individual people score these events higher or lower than they are here.

Life event	"Stress points"
Death of spouse	100
Divorce	73
Marital separation	65
Jail term	63
Death of close family member	63
Personal injury or illness	53
Marriage	50
Being fired at work	47
Marital reconciliation	45
Retirement	45
Change in health of a family member	44
Pregnancy	40
Sex difficulties	39
Gain of new family member	39
Business readjustment	39
Change in financial state	38
Death of close friend	37
Change to different line of work	36
Change in number of arguments with spouse	35
Mortgage over $10,000	31
Foreclosure of mortgage or loan	30
Change in responsibilities at work	29

Source: Reprinted by permission from *Understanding Normal and Clinical Nutrition* by Eleanor Whitney and Corrine Cataldo. Copyright © 1983 by West Publishing Company. All rights reserved. (p. 191).

prarenal glands brings about a wide range of physical changes that are necessary to prepare the body to deal with the impending threat. These changes include increased heart rate and stroke volume, and decreased digestion.

During the **resistance stage,** the body increases its capacity to deal with stress. However, if the stressor continues for a prolonged period of time, the heightened physiological adjustment that is maintained may have a detrimental effect on the body.

Life event	"Stress points"
Son or daughter leaving home	29
Trouble with in-laws	29
Outstanding personal achievement	28
Wife beginning or stopping work	26
School beginning or ending	26
Change in living conditions	25
Revision of personal habits	24
Trouble with boss	23
Change in work hours or conditions	20
Change in residence	20
Change in schools	20
Change in recreation	19
Change in church activities	19
Change in social activities	18
Mortgage or loan less than $10,000	17
Change in sleeping habits	16
Change in number of family get-togethers	15
Change in eating habits	15
Vacation	13
Christmas	12
Minor violations of the law	11

When the body can no longer deal effectively with stress, the **exhaustion stage,** or distress, is evident. The exhaustion stage may manifest itself in high blood pressure, extra heartbeats, and emotional problems.

Determine your behavioral and physiological reactions to stress from tables 12.2 and 12.3. Table 12.4 measures your style of coping with stress. This self-evaluation may help to give you some perspective on developing techniques for stress reduction.

Table 12.2 Behavioral reactions to stress

Circle the number that best represents frequency of occurrence of the following behavioral symptoms and add up the total number of points.

	Never	Infrequently (more than once in six months)	Occasionally (more than once per month)	Very often (more than once per week)	Constantly
1. Difficulty relaxing	1	2	3	4	5
2. Generalized anxiety (no known cause)	1	2	3	4	5
3. Easily angered	1	2	3	4	5
4. Short attention span	1	2	3	4	5
5. Bored	1	2	3	4	5
6. Sexual difficulties or problems	1	2	3	4	5
7. Accident prone	1	2	3	4	5
8. Overeating	1	2	3	4	5
9. Drug usage	1	2	3	4	5
10. Alcohol usage	1	2	3	4	5
11. Inability to control emotions	1	2	3	4	5
12. Inability to concentrate	1	2	3	4	5
13. Distortions in memory	1	2	3	4	5
14. Difficulty in making decisions	1	2	3	4	5
15. Racing thoughts	1	2	3	4	5
16. Pessimistic	1	2	3	4	5
17. Sleeping difficulties	1	2	3	4	5
18. Urge to cry	1	2	3	4	5
19. Blaming others for your anxiety	1	2	3	4	5
20. Frustration	1	2	3	4	5
21. Hostility	1	2	3	4	5
22. Irritability	1	2	3	4	5
23. Impatience	1	2	3	4	5
24. Inflexibility	1	2	3	4	5
25. Powerless	1	2	3	4	5
26. Agitated	1	2	3	4	5
27. Out of control	1	2	3	4	5

Interpretation

40—Low psychological symptoms of stress response
41–60—Moderate psychological symptoms of stress response
61–80—High psychological symptoms of stress response
Over 80—Excessive psychological symptoms of stress response

Source: From *Presidential Sports Award Fitness Manual*, edited by H. Ebel, N. Sol, D. Bailey, and S. Schecter. Copyright © 1983 FitCom Corporation, Havertown, PA.

Table 12.3 Physiological reactions to stress

Circle the number that best represents the frequency of occurrence of the following physical symptoms and add up the total number of points.

	Never	Infrequently (more than once in six months)	Occasionally (more than once per month)	Very often (more than once per week)	Constantly
1. Tension headaches	1	2	3	4	5
2. Migraine (vascular) headaches	1	2	3	4	5
3. Stomachaches	1	2	3	4	5
4. Increase in blood pressure	1	2	3	4	5
5. Cold hands	1	2	3	4	5
6. Acidy stomach	1	2	3	4	5
7. Shallow, rapid breathing	1	2	3	4	5
8. Diarrhea	1	2	3	4	5
9. Palpitations	1	2	3	4	5
10. Shaky hands	1	2	3	4	5
11. Burping	1	2	3	4	5
12. Gassiness	1	2	3	4	5
13. Increased urge to urinate	1	2	3	4	5
14. Sweaty feet/hands	1	2	3	4	5
15. Oily skin	1	2	3	4	5
16. Fatigue/exhausted feeling	1	2	3	4	5
17. Panting	1	2	3	4	5
18. Dry mouth	1	2	3	4	5
19. Hand tremor	1	2	3	4	5
20. Backache	1	2	3	4	5
21. Neck stiffness	1	2	3	4	5
22. Gum chewing	1	2	3	4	5
23. Grinding teeth	1	2	3	4	5
24. Constipation	1	2	3	4	5
25. Tightness in chest or heart	1	2	3	4	5
26. Dizziness	1	2	3	4	5
27. Nausea/vomiting	1	2	3	4	5
28. Menstrual distress	1	2	3	4	5

Source: From *Presidential Sports Award Fitness Manual,* edited by H. Ebel, N. Sol, D. Bailey, and S. Schecter. Copyright © 1983 FitCom Corporation, Havertown, PA.

Table 12.3 Physiological reactions to stress (*Continued*)

	Never	Infrequently (more than once in six months)	Occasionally (more than once per month)	Very often (more than once per week)	Constantly
29. Skin blemishes	1	2	3	4	5
30. Heart pounding	1	2	3	4	5
31. Colitis	1	2	3	4	5
32. Asthma	1	2	3	4	5
33. Indigestion	1	2	3	4	5
34. High blood pressure	1	2	3	4	5
35. Palpitations	1	2	3	4	5
36. Hyperventilation	1	2	3	4	5
37. Arthritis	1	2	3	4	5
38. Skin rash	1	2	3	4	5
39. Bruxism/jaw pain	1	2	3	4	5
40. Allergy	1	2	3	4	5

Interpretation

40–75 Low physiological symptoms of stress response
76–100 Moderate physiological symptoms of stress response
101–150 High physiological symptoms of stress response
Over 150 Excessive physiological symptoms of stress response

Table 12.4 Coping life-style inventory

For each of the items listed, circle the number that best represents what you do when you feel stressed.

	Never	Infrequently (more than once in six months)	Occasionally (more than once per month)	Very often (more than once per week)	Constantly
1. Lose control (e.g., excessive crying)	1	2	3	4	5
2. React on emotions and not intellect	1	2	3	4	5
3. Freeze—controlled by physical symptoms (e.g., shaking)	1	2	3	4	5

Source: From *Presidential Sports Award Fitness Manual*, edited by H. Ebel, N. Sol, D. Bailey, and S. Schecter. Copyright © 1983 FitCom Corporation, Havertown, PA.

Table 12.4 *Continued*

	Never	Infrequently (more than once in six months)	Occasionally (more than once per month)	Very often (more than once per week)	Constantly
4. Use drugs	1	2	3	4	5
5. Use alcohol	1	2	3	4	5
6. Avoid stressor as best I can	1	2	3	4	5
7. Ignore or run from stressor	1	2	3	4	5
8. Internalize feelings (keep inside)	1	2	3	4	5
9. Allow people to take advantage of me	1	2	3	4	5
10. Remain passive because of fear of hurting others	1	2	3	4	5
11. Put off stressful situations until they "come to a head"	1	2	3	4	5
12. Watch television	1	2	3	4	5
13. Read nonprofessional material	1	2	3	4	5
14. Spend time working on hobbies	1	2	3	4	5
15. Binge eat	1	2	3	4	5
16. Listen to music	1	2	3	4	5
17. Face situation head-on	1	2	3	4	5
18. Do something physical (i.e., exercise related)	1	2	3	4	5
19. Ask friends for advice	1	2	3	4	5
20. Get involved with formal relaxation activity	1	2	3	4	5
21. Do yoga, t'ai chi, or meditate	1	2	3	4	5
22. Use positive self-talk (e.g., "Things will work out—I just know it")	1	2	3	4	5
23. Do imagery or fantasy activities	1	2	3	4	5
24. Engage in self-hypnosis	1	2	3	4	5
25. Do nothing (let it be)	1	2	3	4	5
26. Feel the stressor is out of your control	1	2	3	4	5

Table 12.4 Coping life-style inventory (*Continued*)

	Never	Infrequently (more than once in six months)	Occasionally (more than once per month)	Very often (more than once per week)	Constantly
27. Expect the worst to happen	1	2	3	4	5
28. Try to face or attack your fears head-on	1	2	3	4	5
29. Say it's stupid or illogical to get upset	1	2	3	4	5
30. Work out a plan to control stressor	1	2	3	4	5
31. Take out time from daily activities to improve your mental state or well-being	1	2	3	4	5
32. Put off tasks when they aren't important to immediate or future goals	1	2	3	4	5
33. Seek medical help when stress becomes excessive	1	2	3	4	5

Your Style?
This inventory is not intended to judge your coping life-style as good or bad, but rather to make you more aware of what your present style is, so that you can make any adjustments that might be necessary.

Coping Styles
A study of many stress intervention techniques identified the following ten most commonly used styles of coping. Try to identify any that you often use.

1. Lose Control—You freeze, cry excessively, engage in binge eating, or hyperventilate. In other words, your symptoms control you instead of you controlling them. (numbers 1, 2, 3, and 9 on the "Coping Life-Style Inventory")

2. No Active Involvement (Negative)—You feel that stress is out of control and think the worst will probably happen to you. You tell yourself that things won't work out and that there is no reason to try and do anything about it. You are simply pessimistic. (numbers 26, 27)

3. No Active Involvement (Positive)—You don't do anything at all because of your belief that things will work out for the best or that *someone* is watching out for you. You are simply optimistic. (numbers 22 and 25)

4. Divert—You try to distract your mind away from stressful thoughts and emotions. To accomplish this, you might watch television, read books, clean, exercise, work, listen to music, cook, or involve yourself in a hobby. (numbers 12, 13, 14, 15, and 16)

5. Escape—You try to disassociate and run from stressful thoughts and emotions. You might go on vacation, sleep, drink enough alcohol to forget, work long hours, use drugs, and even engage in sexual activity as a means of escaping (numbers 4, 5, 6, and 7)

6. Suppress—You avoid, deny, rationalize, and use any other mental device ("defense mechanism") to protect you from directly facing the stress of daily living. Passive individuals often use suppression as their primary means of coping. (numbers 8 and 11)

7. Active Involvement—This is when you really enter into and attack your problems realistically. Examples of active involvement are when you assert yourself and engage in direct problem solving. In addition, you should set up a schedule of exercise and relaxation. (numbers 17, 18, 19, and 20)

8. Altered State of Confusion—This is when you try to change your frame of mind by getting into activities like imagery, sensory deprivation (isolation tanks), meditation, and self-hypnosis. (numbers 21, 23, and 24)

9. Prevent Stress Reactions—This is really not a coping method. Its objective is to prevent you from experiencing excessive stress by making changes in your life-style and interactions. Examples of preventive coping techniques include time management, cognitive restructuring, fear control training, and taking an occasional day off for "mental health." (numbers 28, 29, 30, 31, and 32)

10. Seek Medical Help—Sometimes, all of the books and self-training programs are not helpful enough, and there is a need to seek additional medical or psychological assistance. This may be a most important coping method under certain circumstances. (number 33)

Your Personality—Type A or Type B?

Research over the past ten years has focused on what is perhaps one of the most critical personal influences on stress. This characteristic was first introduced by Friedman and Rosenman and is called type A personality (as opposed to type B personality). Type A personality is characterized by impatience, restlessness, aggressiveness, competitiveness, and intolerance to frustration. Type A individuals tend to invest long hours on the job to meet pressing and recurring deadlines. Type B people, on the other hand, experience no pressing deadlines or conflicts and are relatively free of any sense of time, urgency, or hostility.

Research indicates that type A individuals are more prone to heart disease and more prone to a second heart attack than type B individuals. However, it is important to remember that a number of other variables are associated with heart disease in addition to your physiological response to stress. Most importantly, keep in mind that it is possible to modify your personality type and subsequent response to stress.

Use figure 12.1 to determine your personality type.

Stress Management

In this section, we discuss six useful ways to turn off stress and also a variety of relaxation techniques that are helpful in stress management. The recommendations that follow are not a panacea for stress but may give you some insight into dealing with it effectively. In the final analysis, however, the best recommendation for dealing with stress is: Know your limits. You must know when your various frustrations, conflicts, and stresses are getting to you and take appropriate action to limit or modify these stresses.

Instructions

Below are fourteen questions relating to you and your life. For each question, please check "Yes", "Sometimes", or "No" to the left of the question in the appropriate boxes. Then score each answer at the far left by assigning a 3 to each "Yes" answer, a 2 to each "Sometimes" answer, and a 1 to each "No" answer.

	Yes	Sometimes	No	
1				When working on a task, do you move rapidly?
2				Do you strive to do everything in the most efficient manner?
3				Can you enjoy doing nothing productive for several hours or days?
4				Do you wait in line patiently, as in a grocery store or bank?
5				Do you do two things at one time, such as read and eat, talk on the phone and do something with your hands?
6				Do you stay relaxed when you have a deadline to meet?
7				Do you get impatient when someone else is slow or inefficient in doing a job?
8				Do you act spontaneously without planning carefully ahead or weighing all the consequences?
9				Do you hurry through routine, repetitive acts, such as washing dishes, making out deposit slips, writing checks?
10				Do you try to hurry other people or tell them how to do things?
11				Do you live pretty much in the present, enjoying the beauty and excitement of everyday life?
12				Do you listen to others talk more than you talk about your own interests?
13				When in a car, do you get impatient or angry with slow or erratic drivers?
14				When you think about your situation in life, are you satisfied with what you have accomplished?

Scoring: Add items 1,2,5,7,9,10, and 13 to determine your type A personality score. Add items 3,4,6,8,11,12, and 14 to determine your type B personality score. There are no norms for this test. However, you may compute the ratio of A/B in a measure of your tendency to a type A profile.

Turning Off Stress

Six ways to turn off stress are:

1. **Try to Change How You Perceive Specific Stress-Inducing Events.** For example, the next time a person in another car does something foolish, try not to perceive him or her as the enemy who is out to run you off the road, but as a friend who has simply made a driving mistake.

2. **Try to Understand and Deal with Your Anger.** Acknowledge your anger to yourself. Learn to differentiate between levels of anger. Try to diagnose the threat that is causing you to be angry—it may be the result of a difference in values or in style and be no real threat to you at all. Finally, try letting go of anger through forgiveness and by canceling the charges against the other person.

3. **Take Time to Relax or Meditate.** Try to manage your time more effectively so that you don't court stress through disorganized scheduling.

4. **Expand Your Social Support System.** Contact and try to establish relationships with new individuals or groups who may be able to give you emotional support.

5. **Regular Exercise Is an Essential Ingredient in Reducing Stress.** Considerable evidence indicates that individuals who regularly exercise have a lower arousal to stress than individuals who are less fit. Exercise aids in balancing and stabilizing the physiological consequences of emotional stress. Exercise also maintains your body systems in a fit state so that they are able to handle effectively any additional stress. Exercise also ensures normal fatigue and relaxation.

6. **Good Nutrition Is Vital.** Eat regular, well-balanced meals, and avoid alcohol and cigarettes.

Figure 12.1 Evaluation of personality type. From *Introduction to Organizational Behavior* by Richard Steers. Copyright © 1981 by Scott, Foresman and Company. Reprinted by permission. (Figure on p. 202)

Relaxation Techniques

There probably are times during the day when you just want to unwind, relax, take time out, and turn off anxiety-producing stimuli. Both psychologically and physiologically, there is a need to relax the tension that is an ever-present companion in all of us. Tension manifests itself in muscle contractions, shallow breathing, clenched jaws, and a variety of other involuntary responses. With a little practice and patience, you can begin to free yourself of tension with such simple relaxation and meditation techniques as the seven-step relaxation program, hatha-yoga, the progressive relaxation exercise, and autogenic training. It is important to relieve the tension in both your body and your brain so that they both relax as one.

Keep in mind, however, that even though relaxation can reduce arousal and be just as effective as exercise in reducing the stress response, it does not bring with it the physiological advantages of rigorous exercise.

The Seven-Step Relaxation Program

1. **Establish a Quiet Environment.**   Arrange for things to be as quiet as possible. Avoid having to answer the phone or door, or respond to other distracting stimuli.
2. **Find a Comfortable Position.**   Sit in a comfortable chair or lie on the floor. The main thing is that you have full body support.
3. **Close Your Eyes.**   Now use your imagination. Place yourself in a relaxing environment, such as a beach or another enjoyable place.
4. **Maintain a Passive Attitude.**   Focus your attention on your bodily sensations. Diffuse your concentration by letting thoughts pass out of your awareness.
5. **Take a Deep Breath.**   Tighten your muscles for a few seconds.
6. **Exhale and Relax.**   Feel the release in tension and the heaviness of your muscles as you exhale and fall into the comfortable position.
7. **Repeat Steps 1–6 Two or Three Times or Until You Are Relaxed.** Take fifteen to twenty minutes to achieve complete relaxation, with about thirty seconds between each phase.

Hatha-Yoga Rest Procedures

The hatha-yoga rest procedures illustrated in figures 12.2 and 12.3 also may be valuable in achieving relaxation and releasing tension.

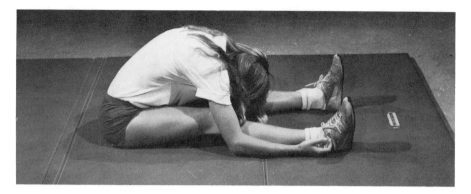

Figure 12.2 Child's pose (darnikasava). Sit on a mat, with your knees together and your feet slightly apart. Bend forward at the groin and stretch your trunk until your forehead rests on the mat. Tuck in your chin slightly to lengthen your neck. Place your hands by your feet, palms up. Relax your entire body. You may place a small pillow between your feet at the buttocks and a small pillow under your head if your head does not touch the floor. Remain in this position for five to ten minutes.

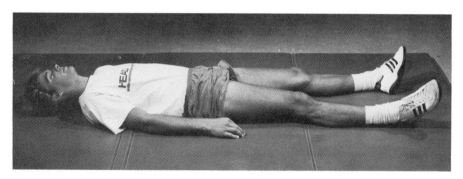

Figure 12.3 Corpse pose (savasana). Lie on your back with your legs straight and your feet about eighteen inches apart, toes falling out. Your hands should be about a foot away from your thighs, palms up. Close your eyes, breathe, and relax with each exhalation. Let your entire body sink toward the earth. Relax all of your muscles. Keep your jaw loose so that your teeth are not touching. Remain in this position for five to twenty minutes. You also may try placing your hands, palms down, across your chest, and bending your knees with your feet on the floor near your buttocks.

The Progressive Relaxation Exercise

The **progressive relaxation exercise** that follows constitutes a more comprehensive muscle relaxation program.

General Instructions

1. The progressive relaxation exercise follows a systematic pattern: right hand (or dominant hand), left hand, right bicep, left bicep, forehead, eyes, facial area, chest, abdomen, and both legs and feet. At the start, repeat the exercise for each group twice before going to the next group. After completing each muscle group, refrain from moving that area so that it remains relaxed.

2. If you are doing the relaxation exercise for the first time, have someone else read the instructions aloud for you to follow.

3. Whoever reads the instructions should do so in a normal voice, pacing the speed by doing the tension exercises. The aim is to tense the muscle group long enough to be noticeable but not long enough to be painful or to lead to cramps or fatigue.

4. Some muscle groups (for example, the eyes, the jaws, and the feet) should be tensed for a shorter span—about three seconds— to avoid pain or cramping.

5. After you have done the exercise once under the direction of someone else, you can practice the exercise alone by simply tensing and relaxing each muscle group in sequence.

6. After three or four practice sessions, omit the muscle-tensing exercises and concentrate simply on having each muscle group become relaxed or limp, again in sequence. With training, you should be able to develop a state of relaxation within five minutes; with more practice, you may be able to establish relaxation control within one minute. Some individuals are able to achieve relaxation while sitting in chairs or riding in vehicles, and can practice it prior to competition. Control in relaxing specific muscle groups is possible with repetition.

7. Repetition of the deep-breath technique (described in the exercise directions that follow) can establish this as a signal for the initiation of relaxation on a quick-reflex basis.

8. Although the relaxation exercise can be used for other forms of training, the directions here are aimed at teaching you how to control muscle groups to achieve relaxation. As with other physical exercise, your success will depend upon how often you practice and your adherence to the exercise steps. Practice the exercise once a day, five times a week. More frequent practice speeds up training.

Directions for the Progressive Relaxation Exercise

Before beginning the progressive relaxation exercise, get into a comfortable position, preferably lying down on your back. You may use a small pillow for your head. Choose a time of day when you will not be disturbed for an hour. Many people practice in the evening since the relaxation achieved is an especially good way of going to sleep at night. The read-aloud directions for the progressive relaxation exercise follow.*

Hands Close your eyes so as not to be distracted by your surroundings. Now tense your right hand into a fist, as tight as you can get it so that you feel the tension . . . really tight, the tighter the better, so that you can really feel the tension. . . . Now relax the hand, let the tension remove itself . . . feel the muscles become loose . . . and notice the contrast between the tension a moment ago and the relaxation, the absence of tension. . . . Allowing the fingers to relax . . . and then the entire right hand.

(Repeat the exercise for the right hand once.)

Now we'll leave the right hand relaxed and focus on the left hand. Tense the left hand by making it into a fist . . . very tight . . . and again notice how that tension feels . . . focus your attention on the muscles as they are tense. . . . All right, now relax the hand, and notice the contrast between the tension of a moment ago and the relaxation. . . . Continue to be aware of the relaxation of the muscles . . . in the fingers . . . and throughout the entire hand.

(Repeat the exercise for the left hand once.)

Arms (Biceps) We'll leave the hands and the fingers relaxed and move to the biceps. In order to tense the biceps, you will be bending the arm at the elbow and tightening the biceps by moving your hand toward your shoulder. Let's start with the right arm.

Bend your right arm at the elbow so that your hand moves toward your shoulder . . . tight. . . . Keep tightening the biceps as hard as you can . . . focusing your attention on the muscle tension. . . . Really notice how that feels. . . . Now relax . . . letting the arm and hand drop back down . . . and noticing the relaxation, the absence of tension. . . . Feel the relaxation as it takes over the upper arm. . . . Notice the feeling of relaxation in the lower arm, the hand, and the fingers.

(Repeat the exercise for the right arm once.)

Now leave the right arm relaxed and move to the left arm. Tense up the left arm by bending it at the elbow . . . really tense, as tense as you can get it . . . and focus your attention on the feelings of tension. . . . Now relax, letting your arm drop back down. . . .

*Used with permission of Suinn, R. M. *Psychology in Sports; Method and Application* pp. 311–312, copyright 1980 Burgess Publishing Co., Minneapolis, MN.

Notice the difference in feeling between the tension and relaxation. . . . Permit the relaxation to take over the entire left arm . . . the upper arm . . . the forearm . . . the hands . . . and fingers.

(Repeat the exercise for the left arm once.)

Forehead We'll leave the hands and the arms comfortably relaxed and move to the forehead. In order to tense up the forehead, you will frown.

All right, I want you to tense the forehead by frowning. . . . Wrinkle up the forehead area . . . very tight . . . and notice how the tension feels. . . . Now relax. . . . Let the wrinkles smooth themselves out. . . . Allow the relaxation to proceed on its own . . . making the forehead smooth and tension free, as though you were passing your hand over a sheet to smooth it out.

(Repeat the exercise for the forehead once.)

Eyes We'll leave the forehead relaxed and move to the eyes. What I want you to do is close your eyes tighter than they are . . . tighter . . . feeling the tension. . . . (Use less time for tension here so as to avoid afterimages). . . . Now relax . . . keeping the eyes comfortably closed . . . noticing the contrast between the tension and the relaxation now.

(Repeat the exercise for the eyes once.)

Facial Area We'll leave the eyes relaxed and go on to the facial area. To tense up the facial area, I want you to clench your jaws. . . . Bite down on your teeth hard now. . . . Really pay attention to the tension in the facial area and jaws. . . . (Use less time for tension here). . . . Now relax. . . . Let the muscles of the jaws become relaxed. . . . Notice the feeling of relaxation across the lips, the jaws, the entire facial area. . . . Just allow the relaxation to take over.

(Repeat the exercise for the facial area once.)

All right, notice the relaxation in the right hand and the fingers . . . and the feeling of relaxation in the forearm and the upper arms. . . . Notice the relaxation that is present in the left hand and the fingers . . . in the forearm. . . . Let the relaxation take over and include the forehead . . . smooth and without tension . . . the eyes . . . the facial area . . . and the lips and the jaws.

Chest All right, we'll now proceed to help the relaxation across the chest. I want you to tense up the chest muscles by taking a deep breath and holding it for a moment. . . . Notice the tension. . . . Now slowly exhale, breathing normally again . . . and notice the chest muscles as they become more and more relaxed.

(Repeat the exercise for the chest once.)

Abdomen Now we'll move to the stomach. I want you to tense your stomach right now . . . very tight. . . . Pay attention to the tension. . . . Now relax . . . letting the feeling of relaxation take over. . . . Notice the difference in the feeling of tension a moment before and the relaxation.

(Repeat the exercise for the abdomen once.)

Legs and Feet Now we'll proceed with the relaxation. To tense your legs and feet, I want you to point your toes downward until you can feel the muscles of your leg tense. . . . Notice the tension. . . . (Maintain the tension for only about three seconds to avoid cramping of the toes or feet). . . . Now relax. . . . Let the relaxation take over. . . . Feel the comfort.

(Repeat the exercise for the legs and feet once.)

All right, simply enjoy the sense of relaxation and comfort across your body . . . feeling loose and relaxed in the hands and fingers . . . comfortable in the forearms and upper arms . . . noticing the relaxed feeling as it includes the forehead . . . the eyes . . . the facial area . . . the lips and the jaws . . . letting the relaxation include the chest . . . the abdomen . . . and both feet.

Now, to further increase the relaxation, I want you to take a deep breath and slowly exhale . . . using your rhythmical deep breathing to deepen the relaxation and to permit you to become as relaxed as you want . . . breathing slowly in and out . . . using your rhythm to achieve whatever level of relaxation you want . . . and in the future you can use this deep-breathing technique to initiate or to deepen the relaxation whenever you want.

All right, that's fine. . . . Now let your breathing continue normally.

Termination of Exercise In a moment, I'll count backward from three to one. When I get to one, you'll feel alert and refreshed . . . no aches or pains. . . . You can retain the relaxed feeling as long as you wish. . . . All right, three . . . more and more alert . . . two . . . no aches or pains . . . and one . . . you can open your eyes.

Autogenic Training

Autogenic training also has been useful in modifying the stress response. Autogenic training emphasizes concentrating on your muscular and involuntary functions, as well as on your mental state, to regulate yourself perceptually, physiologically, mentally, and muscularly. Through autogenic training, for example, you can regulate your heart rate, respiration, and muscle tension. In addition, self-regulation of your mental state allows you to imagine various states of feeling, to visualize concrete and abstract objects, and to experience colors.

Autogenic training involves three phases: (1) the preparation phase, (2) the relaxation phase, and (3) the activation phase.

Preparation Phase
1. Find a comfortable position—lying on your back is the most common.
2. Breathe deeply and concentrate on your depth of breathing.
3. Tighten all of the muscles in your body as hard as you can for a brief second and then relax as completely as possible. Repeat this procedure three times.

Relaxation Phase
4. Think about making one of your arms as heavy as possible—so heavy that it cannot be lifted.
5. Repeat this with the other arm and then with each of your legs, one at a time, and then with your chest muscles and abdominal muscles.
6. Repeat this procedure several times until you feel totally relaxed.
7. Ignore your environment and concentrate on yourself, particularly your body parts.
8. After a few minutes of relaxation, imagine that first one limb and then another are becoming warm. Repeat this several times with all of the muscle groups until you experience a feeling of warmth.

Activation Phase
9. At the end of the relaxation exercise, you will feel relaxed and refreshed. If you fall asleep during the procedure, don't worry about it. Don't be in a hurry to activate yourself. Stay under the "spell" for a while, enjoying the feeling of relaxation. Let the feeling of relaxation reinforce you for the events to come.
10. After several minutes of relaxation or when you desire to become activated, gradually tighten your muscles in the same order that you relaxed them. Imagine a level of activation that you would like to assume while you are tightening the muscles. Once you have achieved a satisfactory level of activation, reintroduce yourself to your daily activities.

Key Terms

Alarm Reaction Stage The first stage of the stress response, during which your body initially reacts to stress

Autogenic Training A stress management technique that emphasizes concentrating on your muscular and involuntary functions, as well as on your mental state, to regulate yourself perceptually, physiologically, mentally, and muscularly

Exhaustion Stage The third stage of the stress response, during which your body can no longer deal effectively with stress

Progressive Relaxation Exercise A stress management technique involving progressive muscle relaxation

Resistance Stage The second stage of the stress response, during which your body increases its capacity to deal with stress

Stress Response A physiological response to stress that results in heightened mental and physical awareness

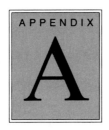

American College of Sports Medicine Position Statement: The Recommended Quantity and Quality of Exercise for Developing and Maintaining Fitness in Healthy Adults

Increasing numbers of persons are becoming involved in endurance training activities, and thus, the need for guidelines for exercise prescription is apparent.

Based on the existing evidence concerning exercise prescription for healthy adults and the need for guidelines, the American College of Sports Medicine makes the following recommendations for the quantity and quality of training for developing and maintaining cardiorespiratory fitness and body composition in the healthy adult:

1. Frequency of training: Three to five days per week.
2. Intensity of training: 60 to 90 percent of maximum heart rate reserve, or 50 to 85 percent of maximum oxygen uptake ($\dot{V}o_2$ max).
3. Duration of training: Fifteen to sixty minutes of continuous aerobic activity. Duration is dependent on the intensity of the activity. Thus, lower-intensity activity should be conducted over a longer period of time. Because of the importance of the "total fitness" effect and the fact that it is more readily attained in longer duration programs, and because of the potential hazards and compliance problems associated with high-intensity activity, lower- to moderate-intensity activity of longer duration is recommended for the nonathletic adult.

Source: Reprinted with permission of the American College of Sports Medicine. Copyright 1978 American College of Sports Medicine.

4. Mode of activity: Any activity that uses large muscle groups, that can be maintained continuously, and that is rhythmical and aerobic in nature, for example, running/jogging, walking/hiking, swimming, skating, bicycling, rowing, cross-country skiing, rope skipping, and various endurance game activities.

Rationale and Research Background

The questions, "How much exercise is enough, and what type of exercise is best for developing and maintaining fitness?" are frequently asked. It is recognized that the term *physical fitness* is composed of a wide variety of variables included in the broad categories of cardiovascular-respiratory fitness, physique and structure, motor function, and many histochemical and biochemical factors. It also is recognized that the adaptive response to training is complex and includes peripheral, central, structural, and functional factors. Although many such variables and their adaptive response to training have been documented, the lack of sufficient in-depth and comparative data relative to frequency, intensity, and duration of training make them inadequate to use as comparative models. Thus, with respect to the previous questions, fitness will be limited to changes in $\dot{V}o_2$ max, total body mass, fat weight (FW), and lean body weight (LBW) factors.

Exercise prescription is based upon the frequency, intensity, and duration of training, the mode of activity (aerobic in nature, for example, listed under no. 4 in the previous list), and the initial level of fitness. In evaluating these factors, the following observations have been derived from studies conducted with endurance training programs.

1. Improvement in $\dot{V}o_2$ max is directly related to frequency (notes 2,23,32,58,59,65,77,79), intensity (notes 2,10,13,26,33,37,42,56,77), and duration (notes 3,14,29,49,56,77,86) of training. Depending upon the quantity and quality of training, improvement in $\dot{V}o_2$ max ranges from 5 to 25 percent (notes 4,13,27,31,35,36,43,45,52,53,62,71,77,78,82,86). Although changes in $\dot{V}o_2$ max greater than 25 percent have been shown, they are usually associated with large total body mass and FW loss, or a low initial level of fitness. Also, as a result of leg fatigue or a lack of motivation, persons with low initial fitness may have spuriously low initial $\dot{V}o_2$ max values.
2. The amount of improvement in $\dot{V}o_2$ max tends to plateau when frequency of training is increased above three days per week (notes 23,62,65). For the nonathlete, there is not enough information available at this time to speculate on the value of

added improvement found in programs that are conducted more than five days per week. Participation of less than two days per week does not show an adequate change in $\dot{V}o_2$ max (notes 24,56,62).

3. Total body mass and FW are generally reduced with endurance training programs (note 67), while LBW remains constant (notes 62,67,87) or increases slightly (note 54). Programs that are conducted at least three days per week (notes 58,59,61,62,87), of at least twenty minutes duration (notes 48,62,87), and of sufficient intensity and duration to expend approximately three-hundred kilocalories (Kcal) per exercise session are suggested as a threshold level for total body mass and FW loss (notes 12,29,62,67). An expenditure of two-hundred Kcal per session has also been shown to be useful in weight reduction if the exercise frequency is at least four days per week (note 80). Programs with less participation generally show little or no change in body composition (notes 19,25,42,62,67,84,85,87). Significant increases in $\dot{V}o_2$ max have been shown with ten to fifteen minutes of high-intensity training (notes 34,49,56,62,77,78). Thus, if total body mass and FW reduction is not a consideration, then short-duration, high-intensity programs may be recommended for healthy, low-risk (cardiovascular disease) persons.

4. The minimal threshold level for improvement in $\dot{V}o_2$ max is approximately 60 percent of the maximum heart rate reserve (50 percent of $\dot{V}o_2$ max) (notes 33,37). Maximum heart rate reserve represents the percent difference between resting and maximum heart rate, added to the resting heart rate. The technique as described by Karvonen, Kentala, and Mustala (note 37), was validated by Davis and Convertino (note 14) and represents a heart rate of approximately 130 to 135 beats/minute for young persons. As a result of the aging curve for maximum heart rate, the absolute heart rate value (threshold level) is inversely related to age and can be as low as 110 to 120 beats/minute for older persons. Initial level of fitness is another important consideration in prescribing exercise (notes 10,40,46,75,77). The person with a low fitness level can get a significant training effect with a sustained training heart rate as low as 110 to 120 beats/minute, while persons of higher fitness levels need a higher threshold of stimulation (note 26).

5. Intensity and duration of training are interrelated, with the total amount of work accomplished being an important factor in improvement in fitness (notes 2,7,12,40,61,62,76,78). Although

more comprehensive inquiry is necessary, present evidence suggests that, when exercise is performed above the minimal threshold of intensity, the total amount of work accomplished is the important factor in fitness development (notes 2,7,12,61,62,76,79) and maintenance (note 68). That is, improvement will be similar for activities performed at a lower intensity/longer duration compared to higher intensity/shorter duration if the total energy costs of the activities are equal.

If frequency, intensity, and duration of training are similar (total Kcal expenditure), the training result appears to be independent of the mode of aerobic activity (notes 56,60,62,64). Therefore, a variety of endurance activities may be used to derive the same training effect.

6. In order to maintain the training effect, exercise must be continued on a regular basis (notes 2,6,11,21,44,73,74). A significant reduction in working capacity occurs after two weeks of detraining (note 73), with participants returning to near pretraining levels of fitness after ten weeks (note 21) to eight months of detraining (note 44). Fifty percent reduction in improvement of cardiorespiratory fitness has been shown after four to twelve weeks of detraining (notes 21,41,73). More investigation is necessary to evaluate the rate of increase and decrease of fitness with varying training loads and reduction in training in relation to level of fitness, age, and length of time in training. Also, more information is needed to better identify the minimal level of work necessary to maintain fitness.

7. Endurance activities that require running and jumping generally cause significantly more debilitating injuries to beginning exercisers than other nonweight-bearing activities (notes 42,55,69). One study showed that beginning joggers had increased foot, leg, and knee injuries when training was performed more than three days per week and longer than thirty minutes duration per exercise session (note 69). Thus, caution should be taken when recommending the type of activity and exercise prescription for the beginning exerciser. Also, the increase of orthopedic injuries as related to overuse (marathon training) with chronic jogger/runners is apparent. Thus, there is a need for more inquiry into the effect that different types of activities and the quantity and quality of training has on short-term and long-term participation.

8. Most of the information concerning training described in this position statement has been conducted on men. The lack of information on women is apparent, but the available evidence indicates that women tend to adapt to endurance training in the same manner as men (notes 8,22,89).

9. Age in itself does not appear to be a deterrent to endurance training. Although some earlier studies showed a lower training effect with middle-aged or elderly participants (notes 4,17,34,83,86), more recent study shows the relative change in $\dot{V}O_2$ max to be similar to younger age groups (notes 3,52,66,75,86). Although more investigation is necessary concerning the rate of improvement in $\dot{V}O_2$ max with age, at present it appears that elderly participants need longer periods of time to adapt to training (notes 17,66). Earlier studies showing moderate to no improvement in $\dot{V}O_2$ max were conducted over a short time span (note 4) or exercise was conducted at a moderate to low Kcal expenditure (note 17), thus making the interpretation of the results difficult.

   Although $\dot{V}O_2$ max decreases with age and total body mass and FW increase with age, evidence suggests that this trend can be altered with endurance training (notes 9,12,38,39,62). Also, five- to ten-year follow-up studies, where participants continued their training at a similar level, showed maintenance of fitness (notes 39,70). A study of older competitive runners showed decreases in $\dot{V}O_2$ max from the fourth to seventh decade of life, but also showed reductions in their training load (note 63). More inquiry into the relationship of long-term training (quantity and quality) for both competitors and noncompetitors and physiological function with increasing age is necessary before more definitive statements can be made.

10. An activity such as weight training should not be considered as a means of training for developing $\dot{V}O_2$ max but has significant value for increasing muscular strength and endurance and LBW (notes 16,24,47,49,88). Recent studies evaluating circuit weight training (weight training conducted almost continuously with moderate weights, using ten to fifteen repetitions per exercise session with fifteen to thirty seconds rest between bouts of activity) showed little to no improvements in working capacity and $\dot{V}O_2$ max (notes 1,24,90).

Despite an abundance of information available concerning the training of the human organism, the lack of standardization of testing protocols and procedures, of methodology in relation to training procedures and experimental design, and of a preciseness in the documentation and reporting of the quantity and quality of training prescribed make interpretation difficult (notes 62,67). Interpretation and comparison of results also are dependent on the initial level of fitness (notes 18,74–76,81), the length of time of the training experiment (notes 20,57,58,61,62), and the specificity of the testing and training (note 64). For example, data from training studies using subjects with varied levels of $\dot{V}o_2$ max, total body mass, and FW have found changes to occur in relation to their initial values (notes 5,15,48,50,51), that is, the lower the initial $\dot{V}o_2$ max, the larger the percent of improvement found, and the higher the FW, the greater the reduction. Also, data evaluating trainability with age, comparison of the different magnitudes and quantities of effort, and comparison of the trainability of men and women may have been influenced by the initial fitness levels.

In view of the fact that improvement in the fitness variables discussed in this position statement continues over many months of training (notes 12,38,39,62), it is reasonable to believe that short-term studies conducted over a few weeks have certain limitations. Middle-aged sedentary and older participants may take several weeks to adapt to the initial rigors of training and thus need a longer adaptation period to get the full benefit from a program. How long a training experiment should be conducted is difficult to determine, but fifteen to twenty weeks may be a good minimum standard. For example, two investigations conducted with middle-aged men who jogged either two or four days per week found both groups to improve in $\dot{V}o_2$ max. Midtest results of the sixteen- and twenty-week programs showed no difference between groups, while subsequent final testing found the four-day-per-week group to improve significantly more (notes 58,59). In a similar study with young college men, no differences in $\dot{V}o_2$ max were found among groups after seven to thirteen weeks of interval training (note 20). These latter findings and those of other investigators point to the limitations in interpreting results from investigations conducted over a short time span (notes 62,67).

In summary, frequency, intensity, and duration of training have been found to be effective stimuli for producing a training effect. In general, the lower the stimuli, the lower the training effect (notes 2,12,13,27,35,46,77,78,90), and the greater the stimuli, the greater the effect (notes 2,12,13,27,58,77,78). It also has been shown that endurance training that is less than two days per week, less than 50 percent of maximum oxygen uptake, and less than ten minutes per day is inadequate for developing and maintaining fitness for healthy adults.

Notes

1. Allen, T. E., R. J. Byrd, and D. P. Smith. Hemodynamic consequences of circuit weight training. *Res Q.* 43(1976):299–306.

2. American College of Sports Medicine. *Guidelines for Graded Exercise Testing and Exercise Prescription.* Philadelphia: Lea & Febiger, 1976.

3. Barry, A. J., J. W. Daly, E. D. R. Pruett, J. R. Steinmetz, H. F. Page, N. C. Birkhead, and K. Rodahl. The effects of physical conditioning on older individuals. I. Work capacity, circulatory-respiratory function, and work electrocardiogram. *J. Gerontol.* 21(1966):182–91.

4. Bensetad, A. M. Trainability of old men. *Acta. Med. Scandinav.* 178(1965):321–27.

5. Boileau, R. A., E. R. Buskirk, D. H. Horstman, J. Mendez, and W. C. Nicholas. Body composition changes in obese and lean men during physical conditioning. *Med. Sci. Sports* 3(1971):183–89.

6. Brynteson, P., and W. E. Sinning. The effects of training frequencies on the retention of cardiovascular fitness. *Med. Sci. Sports* 5(1973):29–33.

7. Burke, E. J., and B. D. Franks. Changes in V̇o₂ max resulting from bicycle training at different intensities holding total mechanical work constant. *Res. Q.* 46(1975):31–37.

8. Burke, E. J. Physiological effects of similar training programs in males and females. *Res. Q.* 48(1977):510–17.

9. Carter, J. E. L., and W. H. Phillips. Structural changes in exercising middle-aged males during a two-year period. *J. Appl. Physiol.* 27(1969):787–94.

10. Crews, T. R., and J. A. Roberts. Effects of interaction of frequency and intensity of training. *Res. Q.* 47(1976):48–55.

11. Cureton, T. K., and E. E. Phillips. Physical fitness changes in middle-aged men attributable to equal eight-week periods of training, nontraining, and retraining. *J. Sports Med. Phys. Fitness* 4(1964):1–7.

12. Cureton, T. K. *The Physiological Effects of Exercise Programs upon Adults.* Springfield, Ill.: Charles C Thomas, 1969.

13. Davies, C. T. M., and A. V. Knibbs. The training stimulus, the effects of intensity, duration, and frequency of effort on maximum aerobic power output. *Int. Z. Angew. Physiol.* 29(1971):299–305.

14. Davis, J. A., and V. A. Convertino. A comparison of heart rate methods for predicting endurance training intensity. *Med. Sci. Sports* 7(1975):295–98.

15. Dempsey, J. A. Anthropometrical observations on obese and nonobese young men undergoing a program of vigorous physical exercise. *Res. Q.* 35(1964):275–87.

16. Delorme, T. L. Restoration of muscle power by heavy resistance exercise. *J. Bone and Joint Surgery* 27(1945):645–67.

17. De Vries, H. A. Physiological effects of an exercise training regimen upon men aged 52 to 88. *J. Gerontol.* 24(1970):325–36.

18. Ekblom, B., P. O. Åstrand, B. Saltin, J. Sternberg, and B. Wallstrom. Effect of training on circulatory response to exercise. *J. Appl. Physiol.* 24(1968):518–28.

19. Flint, M. M., B. L. Drinkwater, and S. M. Horvath. Effects of training on women's response to submaximal exercise. *Med. Sci. Sports* 6(1974):89–94.

20. Fox, E. L., R. L. Bartels, C. E. Billings, R. O'Brien, R. Bason, and D. K. Mathews. Frequency and duration of interval training programs and changes in aerobic power. *J. Appl. Physiol.* 38(1975):481–84.

21. Fringer, M. N., and A. G. Stull. Changes in cardiorespiratory parameters during periods of training and detraining in young female adults. *Med. Sci. Sports* 6(1974):20–25.

22. Getchell, L. H., and J. C. Moore. Physical training: comparative responses of middle-aged adults. *Arch. Phys. Med. Rehab.* 56(1975):250–54.

23. Gettman, L. R., M. L. Pollock, J. L. Durstine, A. Ward, J. Ayres, and A. C. Linnerud. Physiological responses of men to one, three, and five day per week training programs. *Res. Q.* 47(1976):638–46.

24. Gettman, L. R., J. Ayres, M. L. Pollock, J. L. Durstine, and W. Grantham. Physiological effects of circuit strength training and jogging on adult men. *Arch. Phys. Med. Rehab.* In press.

25. Girandola, R. N. Body composition changes in women: Effects of high and low exercise intensity. *Arch. Phys. Med. Rehab.* 57(1976):297–300.

26. Gledhill, N., and R. B. Eynon. The intensity of training. In *Training Scientific Basis and Application,* edited by A. W. Taylor and M. L. Howell. Springfield, Ill.: Charles C Thomas, 1972.

27. Golding, L. Effects of physical training upon total serum cholesterol levels. *Res. Q.* 32(1961):499–505.

28. Goode, R.C., A. Virgin, T. T. Romet, P. Crawford, J. Duffin, T. Pallandi, and Z. Woch. Effects of a short period of physical activity in adolescent boys and girls. *Canad. J. Appl. Sports Sci.* 1(1976):241–50.

29. Gwinup, G. Effect of exercise alone on the weight of obese women. *Arch. Int. Med.* 135(1975):676–80.

30. Hanson, J. S., B. S. Tabakin, A. M. Levy, and W. Nedde. Long-term physical training and cardiovascular dynamics in middle-aged men. *Circ.* 38(1968):783–99.

31. Hartley, L. H., G. Grimby, A. Kilbom, N. J. Nilsson, I. Åstrand, J. Bjure, B. Ekblom, and B. Saltin. Physical training in sedentary middle-aged and older men. *Scand. J. Clin. Lab. Invest.* 24(1969):335–44.

32. Hill, J. S. The effects of frequency of exercise on cardiorespiratory fitness of adult men. Master's Thesis, Univ. of Western Ontario, London, 1969.

33. Hollmann, W., and H. Venrath. Experimentelle Untersuchungen zur bedentung aines trainings unterhalb and oberhalb der dauerbeltz stungsgranze. In *Carl Diem Festschrift,* edited by Korbs. W. u. a. Frankfurt/Wein, 1962.

34. Hollman, W. Changes in the capacity for maximal and continuous effort in relation to age. In *Int. Res. Sport Phys. Ed.,* edited by E. Jokl and E. Simon. Springfield, Ill.: Charles C Thomas, 1964.

35. Huibregtse, W. H., H. H. Hartley, L. R. Jones, W. D. Doolittle, and T. L. Criblez. Improvement of aerobic work capacity following nonstrenuous exercise. *Arch. Env. Health,* 27(1973):12–15.

36. Ismail, A. H., D. Corrigan, and D. F. McLeod. Effect of an eight-month exercise program on selected physiological, biochemical, and audiological variables in adult men. *Brit. J. Sports Med.* 7(1973):230–40.

37. Karvonen, M., K. Kentala, and O. Mustala. The effects of training heart rate: a longitudinal study. *Ann. Med. Exptl. Biol. Fenn.* 35(1957):307–15.

38. Kasch, F. W., W. H. Phillips, J. E. L. Carter, and J. L. Boyer. Cardiovascular changes in middle-aged men during two years of training. *J. Appl. Physiol.* 314(1972):53–57.

39. Kasch, F. W., and J. P. Wallace. Physiological variables during ten years of endurance exercise. *Med. Sci. Sports* 8(1976):5–8.

40. Kearney, J. T., A. G. Stull, J. L. Ewing, and J. W. Strein. Cardiorespiratory responses of sedentary college women as a function of training intensity. *J. Appl. Physiol.* 41(1976):822–25.

41. Kendrick, Z. B., M. L. Pollock, T. N. Hickman, and H. S. Miller. Effects of training and detraining on cardiovascular efficiency. *Amer. Corr. Ther. J.* 25(1971):79–83.

42. Kilbom, A., L. Hartley, B. Saltin, J. Bjure, G. Grimby, and I. Åstrand. Physical training in sedentary middle-aged and older men. *Scand. J. Clin. Lab. Invest.* 24(1969):315–22.

43. Knehr, C. A., D. B. Dill, and W. Neufeld. Training and its effect on men at rest and at work. *Amer. J. Physiol.* 136(1942):148–56.

44. Knuttgen, H. G., L. O. Nordesjo, B. Ollander, and B. Saltin. Physical conditioning through interval training with young male adults. *Med. Sci. Sports* 5(1973):220–26.

45. Mann, G. V., L. H. Garrett, A. Farhi, H. Murray, T. F. Billings, F. Shute, and S. E. Schwarten. Exercise to prevent coronary heart disease. *Amer. J. Med.* 46(1969):12–27.

46. Marigold, E. A. The effect of training at predetermined heart rate levels for sedentary college women. *Med. Sci. Sports* 6(1974):14–19.

47. Mayhew, J. L., and P. M. Gross. Body composition changes in young women with high resistance weight training. *Res. Q.* 45(1974):433–39.

48. Milesis, C. A., M. L. Pollock, M. D. Bah, J. J. Ayres, A. Ward, and A. C. Linnerud. Effects of different durations of training on cardiorespiratory function, body composition, and serum lipids. *Res. Q.* 47(1976):716–25.

49. Misner, J. E., R. A. Boileau, B. H. Massey, and J. H. Mayhew. Alterations in body composition of adult men during selected physical training programs. *J. Amer. Geriatr. Soc.* 22(1974):33–38.

50. Moody, D. L., J. Kollias, and E. R. Buskirk. The effect of a moderate exercise program on body weight and skinfold thickness in overweight college women. *Med. Sci. Sports* 1(1969):75–80.

51. Moody, D. L., J. H. Wilmore, R. N. Girandola, and J. P. Royce. The effects of a jogging program on the body composition of normal and obese high school girls. *Med. Sci. Sports* 4(1972):210–13.

52. Myrhe, L., S. Robinson, A. Brown, and F. Pyke. Paper presented to the American College of Sports Medicine, Albuquerque, New Mexico, 1970.

53. Naughton, J., and F. Nagle. Peak oxygen intake during physical fitness program for middle-aged men. *JAMA* 191(1965):899–901.

54. O'Hara, W., C. Allen, and R. J. Shephard. Loss of body weight and fat during exercise in a cold chamber. *Europ. J. Appl. Physiol.* 37(1977):205–18.

55. Oja, P., P. Teraslinna, T. Partaner, and R. Karava. Feasibility of an eighteen-month physical training program for middle-aged men and its effect on physical fitness. *Am. J. Public Health* 64(1975):459–65.

56. Olree, H. D., B. Corbin, J. Penrod, and C. Smith. Methods of achieving and maintaining physical fitness for prolonged space flight. Final progress rep. to NASA, grant no. NGR-04-002-004, 1969.

57. Oscai, L. B., T. Williams, and B. Hertig. Effects of exercise on blood volume. *J. Appl. Physiol.* 24(1968):622–24.

58. Pollock, M. L., T. K. Cureton, and L. Greninger. Effects of frequency of training on working capacity, cardiovascular function, and body composition of adult men. *Med. Sci. Sports* 1(1969):70–74.

59. Pollock, M. L., J. Tiffany, L. Gettman, R. Janeway, and H. Lofland. Effects of frequency of training on serum lipids, cardiovascular function, and body composition. In *Exercise and Fitness,* edited by B. D. Franks. Chicago: Athletic Institute, 1969.

60. Pollock, M. L., H. Miller, R. Janeway, A. C. Linnerud, B. Robertson, and R. Valentino. Effects of walking on body composition and cardiovascular function of middle-aged men. *J. Appl. Physiol.* 30(1971):126–30.

61. Pollock, M. L., J. Broida, Z. Kendrick, H. S. Miller, R. Janeway, and A. C. Linnerud. Effects of training two days per week at different intensities on middle-aged men. *Med. Sci. Sports* 4(1972):192–97.

62. Pollock, M. L. The quantification of endurance training programs. In *Exercise and Sport Sciences Reviews*, edited by J. Wilmore. New York: Academic Press, 1973.

63. Pollock, M. L., H. S. Miller, Jr., and J. Wilmore. Physiological characteristics of champion American track athletes forty to seventy years of age. *J. Gerontol.* 29(1974):645–49.

64. Pollock, M. L., J. Dimmick, H. S. Miller, Z. Kendrick, and A. C. Linnerud. Effects of mode of training on cardiovascular function and body composition of middle-aged men. *Med. Sci. Sports* 7(1975):139–45.

65. Pollock, M. L., H. S. Miller, A. C. Linnerud, and K. H. Cooper. Frequency of training as a determinant for improvement in cardiovascular function and body composition of middle-aged men. *Arch. Phys. Med. Rehab.* 56(1975):141–45.

66. Pollock, M. L., G. A. Dawson, H. S. Miller, Jr., A. Ward, D. Cooper, W. Headly, A. C. Linnerud, and M. M. Nomeir. Physiologic response of men forty-nine to sixty-five years of age to endurance training. *J. Amer. Geriatr. Soc.* 24(1976):97–104.

67. Pollock, M. L., and A. Jackson. Body composition: Measurement and changes resulting from physical training. Proceedings National College Physical Education Association for Men and Women, January 1977, pp. 125–37.

68. Pollock, M. L., J. Ayres, and A. Ward. Cardiorespiratory fitness: Response to differing intensities and durations of training. *Arch. Phys. Med. Rehab.* 58(1977):467–73.

69. Pollock, M. L., L. R. Gettman, C. A. Milesis, M. D. Bah, J. L. Durstine, and R. B. Johnson. Effects of frequency and duration of training on attrition and incidence of injury. *Med. Sci. Sports* 9(1977):31–36.

70. Pollock, M. L., H. S. Miller, and P. M. Ribisl. Body composition and cardiorespiratory fitness in former athletes. *Phys. Sports Med.* In press, 1978.

71. Ribisl, P. M. Effects of training upon the maximal oxygen uptake of middle-aged men. *Int. Z. Angew. Physiol.* 26(1969):272–78.

72. Robinson, S., and P. M. Harmon. Lactic acid mechanism and certain properties of blood in relation to training. *Amer. J. Physiol.* 132(1941):757–69.

73. Roskamm, H. Optimum patterns of exercise for healthy adults. *Canad. Med. Ass. J.* 96(1967):895–99.

74. Saltin, B., G. Blomqvist, J. Mitchell, R. L. Johnson, K. Wildenthal, and C. B. Chapman. Response to exercise after bed rest and after training. *Circ.* 37 and 38, supp. 7, 1–78, 1968.

75. Saltin, B., L. Hartley, A. Kilbom, and I. Åstrand. Physical training in sedentary middle-aged and older men. *Scand. J. Clin. Lab. Invest.* 24(1969):323–34.

76. Sharkey, B. J. Intensity and duration of training and the development of cardiorespiratory endurance. *Med. Sci. Sports* 2(1970):197–202.

77. Shephard, R. J. Intensity, duration, and frequency of exercise as determinants of the response to a training regime. *Int. Z. Angew. Physiol.* 26(1969):272–78.

78. Shephard, R. J. Future research on the quantifying of endurance training. *J. Human Ergology* 3(1975):163–81.

79. Sidney, K. H., R. B. Eynon, and D. A. Cunningham. Effect of frequency of training of exercise upon physical working performance and selected variables representative of cardiorespiratory fitness. In *Training Scientific Basis and Application*, edited by A. W. Taylor. Springfield, Ill.: Charles C Thomas, 1972.

80. Sidney, K. H., R. J. Shephard, and J. Harrison. Endurance training and body composition of the elderly. *Amer. J. Clin. Nutr.* 30(1977):326–33.

81. Siegel, W., G. Blomqvist, and J. H. Mitchell. Effects of a quantitated physical training program on middle-aged sedentary males. *Circ.* 41(1970):19.

82. Skinner, J., J. Holloszy, and T. Cureton. Effects of a program of endurance exercise on physical work capacity and anthropometric measurements of fifteen middle-aged men. *Amer. J. Cardiol.* 14(1964):747–52.

83. Skinner, J. The cardiovascular system with aging and exercise. In *Physical Activity and Aging,* edited by D. Brunner and E. Jokl. Baltimore: University Park Press, 1970.

84. Smith, D. P., and F. W. Stranksy. The effects of training and detraining on the body composition and cardiovascular response of young women to exercise. *J. Sports Med.* 16(1976):112–20.

85. Terjung, R. L., K. M. Baldwin, J. Cooksey, B. Samson, and R. A. Sutter. Cardiovascular adaptation to twelve minutes of mild daily exercise in middle-aged sedentary men. *J. Amer. Geriatr. Soc.* 21(1973):164–68.

86. Wilmore, J. H., J. Royce, R. N. Girandola, F. I. Katch, and V. L. Katch. Physiological alterations resulting from a ten-week jogging program. *Med. Sci. Sports* 2, no. 1(1970):7–14.

87. Wilmore, J. H., J. Royce, R. N. Girandola, F. I. Katch, and V. L. Katch. Body composition changes with a ten-week jogging program. *Med. Sci. Sports* 2(1970):113–17.

88. Wilmore, J. H. Alterations in strength, body composition, and anthropometric measurements consequent in a ten-week weight training program. *Med. Sci. Sports* 6(1974):133–38.

89. Wilmore, J. Inferiority of female athletes: Myth or reality. *J. Sports Med.* 3(1974):1–6.

90. Wilmore, J., R. B. Parr, P. A. Vodak, T. J. Barstow, T. V. Pipes, A. Ward, and P. Leslie. Strength, endurance, BMR, and body composition changes with circuit weight training. Abstract. *Med. Sci. Sports* 8(1976):58–60.

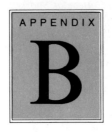

APPENDIX

B

Record Sheets

Record Sheet B–1 Daily exercise program

Name _____   Date _____

Exercise

Fitness level _____

Flexibility	Repetitions
Achilles tendon stretch	
Back stretch	
Groin stretch	
Quadriceps stretch	
Abdominal stretch	
Lower-back stretch	
Upper-trunk stretch	

Fitness level _____

Floor exercise	Repetitions
Modified push-up	
Full push-up	
Head-and-shoulder curl	
Bent-knee sit-up	

Fitness level _____

Strength	RM	Repetitions	Sets
Zottman curl			
Bent-arm lateral			
Heel raise			
Bent-over rowing			
Lateral arm raise			
Standing overhead press			
Bent-arm pullover			
Bench press			
Biceps curl			

Fitness level _____

Cardiovascular	Distance	Duration	Heart rate training effect level
Jogging			
Swimming			
Bicycling			
Walking			
Rope jumping			
Other			

Record Sheet B–2 Flexibility and floor exercise record

			Achilles tendon stretch	Back stretch	Groin stretch	Quadriceps stretch	Abdominal stretch	Upper-trunk stretch	Lower-back stretch	Modified push-up	Full push-up	Head-and-shoulder curl	Bent-knee sit-up
Week	Day	Repetition											

Name _____

Record Sheet B-3 Aerobic exercise record

Name _____

Week	Day	Exercise	Heart rate training effect level	Distance	Duration

Record Sheet B-4 Weight-training record

Exercise	Date					Date				
	RM	Rep.	Set 1	Set 2	Set 3	RM	Rep.	Set 1	Set 2	Set 3

Record Sheet B-5 Circuit-training record

Exercise	Date _____ I Repetitions completed	Date _____ II Repetitions completed	Date _____ III Repetitions completed	Date _____ IV Repetitions completed
1				
2				
3				
4				
5				
6				
7				
8				
9				
10				
11				
12				
13				
14				
15				
16				
17				
18				
19				
20				
Target time				
Actual circuit time				
Postcircuit heart rate				

Record Sheet B-6 Strength record

Name _____

Week	Day	RM Repetition	Zottman curl	Bent-arm lateral	Bent-over rowing	Lateral arm raise	Standing overhead press	Bent-arm pullover	Bench press	Biceps curl	Heel raise	

Record Sheet B-7 Weight-reducing record

Name _____ Date _____

1. Determine your individual caloric allowance, see pp. 136–37.   _____ KCal

2. Determine your percentage of body fat (chapter 3): _____

3. Weight = _____

Percentage of body fat _____ × Body weight _____ = Total fat _____ lbs

Body weight _____ − Total fat _____ = Lean body weight _____

   y = Desired weight   Desired body fat = _____%

y − (y ×Percentage of desired body fat _____) = Body weight _____ −
                                                        (Body weight _____ ×
                                                        Percentage of body fat _____)

        Body Weight _____ − y _____ = Weight loss required _____

Source: Preventive Medicine Center, Weight Control, Palo Alto, CA, 1978.

Record Sheet B-8 Daily caloric intake

Date _____   Weight _____

                                      Percentage of body fat _____

Day	Food	Portion	Calories (from Appendix C)
Breakfast			
Lunch			
Dinner			
Desserts			
Snacks			
Drinks			
Other			

                      Total caloric intake   _____

               Total caloric expenditures   _____
        (from tables 9.5, 9.7–9.10, and Appendix D)

            Caloric difference (positive or negative)   _____

Record Sheet B-9 Caloric record

Name _____

Week	Day	Total caloric intake	Exercise	Caloric expenditure	Weight

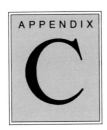

APPENDIX

C

Calorie Counting

Table C-1 Caloric content of food groups

Milk and milk products

	Amount	Calories
Milk, pasteurized, whole	1 cup	165
Milk, canned, evaporated, unsweetened	½ cup	140
Milk, condensed, sweetened	½ cup	480
Milk, nonfat	1 cup	80
Skim milk	1 cup	86
Goat's milk	½ cup	71
Buttermilk, cultured	1 cup	80
Ice cream	1/6 quart	200
Cream, light	1 teaspoon	30
Cream, heavy or whipping	1 teaspoon	50
Cheddar cheese	1 square	115
Cottage cheese	½ cup	100
Cream cheese	2 tablespoons	100
Parmesan cheese	2 teaspoons	110
Roquefort cheese	2 teaspoons	105
Swiss cheese	2 teaspoons	105

Meat, fish, poultry, eggs, nuts

	Amount	Calories
Bacon, medium fat, cooked	3 strips	150
Beef, medium fat, hamburger cooked	¼ pound	225
Chicken, fried	¼ pound	275
Chicken, broiled	quarter chicken	332
Chicken liver	¼ pound	85
Corned beef, canned	4 ounces	240
Frankfurter	1	124
Ham, broiled	¼ pound	300
Ham, smoked, cooked	¼ pound	400
Ham, canned, spiced	¼ pound	290

Table C-1 Caloric content of food groups (*Continued*)

Meat, fish, poultry, eggs, nuts

	Amount	Calories
Lamb, medium fat, leg roast, cooked	¼ pound	270
Lamb, rib chop, cooked	¼ pound	140
Liver (beef)	1 slice	85
Pork, medium fat	¼ pound	365
Pork loin or chops, cooked	1 chop	265
Rib roast, cooked	2 slices (lean to fat)	200 to 400
Rump, cooked	2 slices	190
Sirloin, cooked	¼ pound (lean to fat)	200 to 300
Turkey, medium fat	¼ pound	270
Veal, medium fat, cutlet	¼ pound	220
Veal, medium fat, roast	¼ pound	360
Venison	¼ pound	140
Clams, long and round	¼ pound	80
Cod	1 piece	70
Crab, canned or cooked, meat only	½ cup	85
Flounder	¼ pound	200
Halibut	¼ pound	200
Lobsters	1 (¾ pound)	300
Oysters	5 to 8 medium	80
Salmon, Pacific, cooked	¼ pound	180
Salmon, canned	½ cup	190
Sardines, canned in oil	5 medium	180
Scallops, fried	5 to 6 medium	425
Shrimps, canned, drained	10 to 12 medium	45
Trout	¼ pound (brook/lake)	210 to 290
Tuna	3 ounces	247
Eggs, whole	1 medium	75
Egg white, raw	1 medium	15
Egg yolk, raw	1 medium	60
Almonds, salted	15	100
Brazil nuts	5	100
Cashews, roasted or cooked	10	200
Chestnuts	2 large	200
Peanuts, roasted	½ cup	440
Pecans	1 teaspoon	52
Walnuts	2 teaspoon	95

Soup

Bean soup	1 cup	260
Beef soup	1 cup	115
Beef soup with vegetables	1 cup	80
Chicken noodle soup	1 cup	68
Lentil soup	1 cup	600
Pea soup, creamed	1 cup	270
Tomato soup	1 cup	100
Vegetable soup	1 cup	90

Fruits, fruit juices, and vegetables

	Amount	Calories
Apples	1 sweet	60 to 90
Apple juice, fresh	1 cup	120
Apple sauce, sweetened	½ cup	80
Apricots	1 medium	18
Avocados, fresh	½	279
Bananas	1 (about 6 inches)	88
Blackberries, fresh	½ cup	40
Blackberries, canned, sweetened	½ cup	85
Blueberries, fresh	½ cup	45
Blueberries, canned, sweetened	½ cup	110
Cantaloupe, fresh	½	40
Cherries, canned, sweetened	½ cup	100
Cranberry sauce	2 teaspoons	60
Dates, dried	5 pitted	100
Fruit cocktail, canned	½ cup	80
Grapes, fresh	½ cup	65
Grape juice	½ cup	75
Grapefruit	½ (4 ¼-inch diameter)	75
Grapefruit juice, fresh	½ cup	45
Lemons, fresh	1 (2-inch diameter)	25
Limes, fresh	1	25
Olives, green	2 medium	15
Oranges, fresh	1 (3-inch diameter)	70
Orange juice, fresh	½ cup	55
Peaches, fresh	1 medium	45
Peaches, canned, sweetened	2 halves	85
Pears	1 (2 ½-inch diameter)	95
Pineapple, canned, sweetened	1 cup	200
Pineapple juice, canned	1 cup	120
Plums	1 (2-inch diameter)	30
Prunes, dried, uncooked	4 large	121
Raisins, dried	½ cup	190
Raspberries, fresh	½ cup	50
Raspberries, canned, sweetened	1 cup	100
Strawberries, fresh	10 large	35
Strawberries, frozen, sweetened	½ cup	125
Beans, kidney	½ cup	90
Beans, lima, fresh	½ cup	90
Beans, lima, canned	½ cup	95
Beans, snap, fresh	1 cup	35
Beans, wax, canned	½ cup	20
Beets (beetroots), peeled, fresh	½ cup	34
Broccoli, fresh	½ cup	22
Brussels spouts, fresh	½ cup	30
Cabbage, fresh	Wedge	25
Carrots, canned	½ cup	30
Carrots, fresh	1 (6 inches)	20
Cauliflower, fresh	½ cup	30
Celery	2 stalks	17

Table C-1 Caloric content of food groups (*Continued*)

Fruits, fruit juices, and vegetables

	Amount	Calories
Corn, fresh	1 ear with butter	90
Corn, canned	½ cup	70
Cucumbers	½ (7½ inches)	20
Eggplant, fresh	½ cup	25
Kale, fresh	1 cup	40
Lentils	½ cup	110
Lettuce, fresh	½ head	15
Mushrooms (field)	½ cup	20
Onions	1 (2 ½-inch diameter)	40
Peas, green, fresh	½ cup	60
Peas, canned	½ cup	70
Peppers, green, fresh	1 large	24
Potato chips	7 to 10	110
Potatoes, raw	1 medium	90
Potatoes, french fried	20 pieces	275
Radishes, fresh	4 small	4
Rhubarb, fresh	½ cup	10
Spinach, canned	½ cup	25
Sweet potatoes, fresh	1 small	150
Sweet potatoes, candied	1 medium	300
Sweet potatoes, canned	½ cup	120
Tomatoes, fresh	1 medium	30
Tomatoes, canned	½ cup	25
Tomato catsup	2 teaspoons	40
Tomato juice, canned	½ cup	25

Breads, flour, cereals

	Amount	Calories
Brown bread, enriched	1 slice	100
Corn muffins, enriched	2	220
French bread	1 slice	70
Raisin bread, enriched	1 slice	65
Rye bread, American	1 slice	55
White bread, enriched	1 slice	63
Whole wheat bread	1 slice	55
Cornflakes	1 cup	100
Graham crackers	2	60
Saltine crackers	2	30
Soda crackers	10 small	40
Flour	1 cup	401
Macaroni, cooked	½ cup	70
Noodles, cooked	½ cup	54
Oatmeal, cooked	1 cup	75
Pancakes, wheat	2	150
Pie	1 slice	300 to 400
Popcorn, popped	1 cup	60
Pretzel sticks	15 small	15
Rice, cooked	½ cup	75
Spaghetti, cooked	1 cup	220
Sweet rolls	1	175
Tapioca, cooked	½ cup	130
Waffles, baked	1	225
Wheat germ	1 cup	365

Fats, sweets, alcohol

	Amount	Calories
Butter or margarine	1 teaspoon	100
Mayonnaise	1 teaspoon	100
Olive oil	1 teaspoon	125
Peanut butter	1 teaspoon	85
Salad dressing (French, thousand island)	1 teaspoon	60 to 100
Chocolate, sweetened	2 ½ ounces	335
Chocolate, milk	4 ounces	542
Chocolate, plain	4 ounces	471
Chocolate creams	2	110
Fudge	1 piece	120
Honey	1 teaspoon	65
Jams	1 teaspoon	55
Jellies	1 teaspoon	50
Jelly beans	10 pieces	70
Molasses	1 teaspoon	150
Sugar, maple	1 teaspoon	55
Sugar, cane or beet	1 teaspoon	50
Syrup (corn)	½ cup	427
Beer	1 cup	115
Brandy	1 ounce	70
Eggnog	½ cup	335
Highball	1 cup	165
Port, vermouth, muscatel	½ cup	155
Rum	1 jigger (1 ½ ounces)	140
Whiskey	1 jigger (1 ½ ounces)	130
Wine, white, rosé	½ cup	85 to 105
Carbonated soft drinks	1 cup	80
Chocolate milk	1 cup	250
Cocoa	1 cup	175
Coffee, black	1 cup	1
Coffee with cream and sugar (1 teaspoon each)	1 cup	45
Tea	1 cup	0

Big-calorie culprits

Chocolate milk	1 cup	250
Chocolate candy	3 ounces	453
Chocolate creams	2 ounces	220
Malted milk	1 cup	281
Nuts, cashews	2 ounces	328
Soda with ice cream	1 glass	325
Sundae, chocolate, with 2 teaspoons of syrup	½ cup	330
Whipping cream	1 teaspoon	50

Popular fast foods

Jack-in-the-Box

Hamburger	1	263
Cheeseburger	1	310
French fries	1 serving	270
Onion rings	1 serving	351
French toast	1 serving	537
Pancakes	1 serving	626
Scrambled eggs	1 serving	719

Table C-1 Caloric content of food groups (*Continued*)

Popular fast foods

	Amount	Calories
Kentucky Fried Chicken		
Wing and thigh	1 dinner	661
Drumstick and thigh	1 dinner	643
Wing and thigh, extra crispy	1 dinner	812
Drumstick and thigh, extra crispy	1 dinner	765
McDonald's		
Hotcakes with butter and syrup	1 serving	500
Big Mac	1	563
Quarter pounder	1	424
Regular fries	1 serving	220
Chocolate shake	1	383
Taco Bell		
Beef burrito	1 serving	466
Burrito supreme	1 serving	457
Enchirito	1 serving	454
Wendy's		
Single hamburger	1 serving	470
Double hamburger	1 serving	670
Triple hamburger	1 serving	850
Double hamburger with cheese	1 serving	800
French fries	1 serving	330
Frosty	1	390

Table C-2 Energy values for common snack foods

	Amount or average serving	Energy (in Kcal)
"Just a little sandwich"		
Hamburger on bun	3-inch patty	330
Peanut butter sandwich	2 tablespoons peanut butter	330
Cheese sandwich	1 ounce cheese	280
Ham sandwich	1 ounce ham	320
TV snack		
Pizza (cheese)	⅛ of 14-inch diameter pie	185
Popcorn with oil and salt	1 cup	40
Pretzel, thin, twisted	1	25
Cheese fondue	½ cup	265
Dips (sour cream)	½ cup	248
Chippers	10	150
Beverages		
Carbonated drinks, soda, root beer, etc.	6 ounces	80
Cola beverages	12 ounces	150
Club soda	8 ounces	5
Chocolate malted milk	10 ounces	500
Ginger ale	6 ounces	60
Tea or coffee, straight	1 cup	0
Tea or coffee, with 2 tablespoons cream and 2 teaspoons sugar	1 cup	90

Source: From *Health and Physical Fitness* by William P. Marley. Copyright © 1982 by CBS College Publishing. *Reprinted by permission.*

Table C–2 (*Continued*)

	Amount or average serving	Energy (in Kcal)
Alcoholic drinks		
Ale	8 ounces	155
Beer	8 ounces	110
Highball (with ginger ale—ladies' style)	8 ounces	185
Manhattan	Average	165
Martini	Average	140
Wine, muscatel, or port	2 ounces	95
Sherry	2 ounces	75
Scotch, bourbon, rye	1½-ounce jigger	130
Fruits		
Apple	1 (3-inch diameter)	75
Banana	1 (6 inches)	130
Grapes	30 medium	75
Orange	1 (2¾-inch diameter)	70
Pear	1	65
Salted nuts		
Almonds, filberts, hazelnuts	12 to 15	95
Cashews	6 to 8	90
Peanuts	15 to 17	85
Pecans, walnuts	10 to 15 halves	100
Candies		
Chocolate bars,		
Plain, sweet milk	1 bar (1 ounce)	155
With almonds	1 bar (1 ounce)	140
Chocolate-covered bar	1 bar	270
Chocolate cream, bonbon, fudge	1 piece, 1-inch square	90 to 120
Caramels, plain	2 medium	85
Hard candies, Lifesaver type	1 roll	95
Peanut brittle	1 piece (2½-inch square)	110
Desserts		
Pie		
Fruit—apple, etc.	1/6 pie, 1 average serving	410
Custard	1/6 pie, 1 average serving	265
Mince	1/6 pie, 1 average serving	400
Pumpkin pie with whipped cream	1/6 pie, 1 average serving	460
Cake		
Chocolate layer	3-inch section	350
Doughnut, sugared	1 average	150
Sweets		
Ice cream		
Plain vanilla	1/6 quart	200
Chocolate and other flavors	1/6 quart	260
Orange sherbert	½ cup	120
Sundaes, small chocolate nut with whipped cream	Average	400
Ice-cream sodas, chocolate	10 ounces	270
Midnight snacks for icebox raiders		
Cold potato	½ medium	65
Chicken leg (fried)	1 average	88
Milk	7 ounces	140
Mouthful of roast	½ inch × 2 inches × 3 inches	130
Piece of cheese	¼ inch × 2 inches × 3 inches	120
Leftover beans	½ cup	105
Brownie	¾ inch × 1¾ inches × 2¼ inches	140
Cream puff	4-inch diameter	450

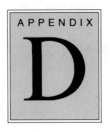

APPENDIX

D

Calorie Expenditure per Minute for Various Activities

Appendix D Calorie expenditure per minute for various activities

Body weight	90	99	108	117	125	134	143	152	161	170	178	187	196	205	213	222	231	240	249	257	266	275
Archery	3.1	3.4	3.7	4.0	4.5	4.6	4.9	5.2	5.5	5.8	6.1	6.4	6.7	7.0	7.3	7.6	7.9	8.2	8.5	8.8	9.1	9.4
Badminton (recreation)	3.4	3.8	4.1	4.4	4.8	5.1	5.4	5.6	6.1	6.4	6.8	7.1	7.4	7.8	8.1	8.3	8.8	9.1	9.4	9.8	10.1	10.4
Badminton (competition)	5.9	6.4	7.0	7.6	8.1	8.7	9.3	9.9	10.4	11.0	11.6	12.1	12.7	13.3	13.9	14.4	15.0	15.6	16.1	16.7	17.3	17.9
Baseball (player)	2.8	3.1	3.4	3.6	3.9	4.2	4.5	4.7	5.0	5.3	5.5	5.8	6.1	6.4	6.6	6.9	7.2	7.5	7.7	8.0	8.3	8.6
Baseball (pitcher)	3.5	3.9	4.3	4.6	5.0	5.3	5.7	6.0	6.4	6.7	7.1	7.4	7.8	8.1	8.5	8.8	9.2	9.5	9.9	10.2	10.6	10.9
Basketball (half-court)	2.5	3.3	3.5	3.8	4.1	4.4	4.7	4.9	5.3	5.6	5.9	6.2	6.4	6.7	7.0	7.3	7.5	7.6	8.2	8.5	8.8	9.0
Basketball (moderate)	4.2	4.6	5.0	5.5	5.9	6.3	6.7	7.1	7.5	7.9	8.3	8.8	9.2	9.6	10.0	10.4	10.8	11.2	11.6	12.1	12.5	12.9
Basketball (competition)	5.9	6.5	7.1	7.7	8.2	8.8	9.4	10.0	10.6	11.1	11.7	12.3	12.9	13.5	14.0	14.6	15.0	15.2	16.3	16.9	17.5	18.1
Bicycling (level) 5.5 MPH	3.0	3.3	3.6	3.9	4.2	4.5	4.8	5.1	5.4	5.6	5.9	6.2	6.5	6.8	7.1	7.4	7.7	8.0	8.3	8.6	8.9	9.2
Bicycling (level) 13 MPH	6.4	7.1	7.7	8.3	8.9	9.6	10.2	10.8	11.4	12.1	12.7	13.4	14.0	14.6	15.2	15.9	16.5	17.1	17.8	18.4	19.0	19.6
Bowling (nonstop)	4.0	4.4	4.8	5.2	5.6	5.9	6.3	6.7	7.1	7.5	7.9	8.3	8.7	9.1	9.5	9.8	10.2	10.6	11.0	11.4	11.8	12.2
Boxing (sparring)	3.0	3.3	3.6	3.9	4.2	4.5	4.8	5.1	5.4	5.6	5.9	6.2	6.5	6.8	7.1	7.4	7.7	8.0	8.3	8.6	8.9	9.2
Calisthenics	3.0	3.3	3.6	3.9	4.2	4.5	4.8	5.1	5.4	5.6	5.9	6.2	6.5	6.8	7.1	7.4	7.7	8.0	8.3	8.6	8.9	9.2
Canoeing, 2.5 MPH	1.8	1.9	2.0	2.2	2.3	2.5	2.7	3.0	3.2	3.4	3.6	3.7	3.9	4.1	4.3	4.4	4.6	4.8	5.0	5.1	5.3	5.5
Canoeing, 4.0 MPH	4.2	4.6	5.0	5.5	5.9	6.3	6.7	7.1	7.5	7.9	8.3	8.7	9.2	9.4	10.0	10.5	10.8	11.2	11.6	12.0	12.4	12.9
Dance, modern (moderate)	2.5	2.8	3.0	3.2	3.5	3.7	4.0	4.2	4.5	4.7	5.0	5.2	5.4	5.7	5.9	6.2	6.4	6.7	6.9	7.2	7.4	7.6
Dance, modern (vigorous)	3.4	3.7	4.1	4.4	4.7	5.1	5.4	5.7	6.1	6.4	6.7	7.1	7.4	7.7	8.1	8.4	8.7	9.1	9.4	9.7	10.1	10.4
Dance, fox-trot	2.7	2.9	3.2	3.4	3.7	4.0	4.2	4.5	4.7	5.0	5.3	5.5	5.8	6.0	6.3	6.6	6.8	7.1	7.3	7.6	7.9	8.1
Dance, rumba	4.2	4.6	5.0	5.4	5.8	6.2	6.6	7.0	7.4	7.8	8.2	8.6	9.0	9.4	9.8	10.2	10.6	11.0	11.5	11.9	12.3	12.6
Dance, square	4.1	4.5	4.9	5.3	5.7	6.1	6.5	6.9	7.3	7.8	8.1	8.5	8.9	9.3	9.7	10.1	10.5	10.9	11.3	11.7	12.1	12.4
Dance, waltz	3.1	3.4	3.7	4.0	4.3	4.6	4.9	5.2	5.5	5.8	6.1	6.4	6.7	7.0	7.3	7.6	7.9	8.2	8.5	8.8	9.1	9.4

Source: From *Physiological Measurement of Metabolic Functions in Man* by C. Frank Consolazio, Robert E. Johnson, and Louis J. Pecora, pp. 331–332. Copyright 1963 McGraw-Hill Book Company. Reprinted by permission of the publisher.

Appendix D—*Continued*

Body weight	90	99	108	117	125	134	143	152	161	170	178	187	196	205	213	222	231	240	249	257	266	275
Fencing (moderate)	3.0	3.3	3.6	3.9	4.2	4.5	4.8	5.1	5.4	5.6	6.0	6.2	6.5	6.8	7.1	7.4	7.7	8.0	8.3	8.6	8.9	9.2
Fencing (vigorous)	6.2	6.8	7.4	8.0	8.6	9.2	9.8	10.4	11.0	11.6	12.2	12.8	13.4	14.0	14.6	15.2	15.8	16.4	17.0	17.6	18.2	18.8
Football (moderate)	3.0	3.3	3.6	4.0	4.2	4.5	4.8	5.1	5.4	5.7	6.0	6.2	6.5	6.8	7.1	7.4	7.7	8.0	8.3	8.6	8.9	9.2
Football (vigorous)	5.0	5.5	6.0	6.4	6.9	7.4	7.9	8.4	8.9	9.4	9.8	10.3	10.8	11.3	11.8	12.3	12.8	13.2	13.7	14.2	14.7	15.2
Golf, twosome	3.3	3.6	3.9	4.2	4.5	4.8	5.2	5.5	5.8	6.1	6.4	6.7	7.1	7.4	7.7	8.0	8.3	8.6	9.0	9.3	9.6	10.0
Golf, foursome	2.4	2.7	2.9	3.2	3.4	3.6	3.9	4.1	4.3	4.6	4.8	5.1	5.3	5.5	5.8	6.0	6.2	6.5	6.7	7.0	7.2	7.4
Handball	5.9	6.4	7.0	7.6	8.1	8.7	9.3	9.9	10.4	11.0	11.6	12.1	12.7	13.3	13.9	14.4	15.0	15.6	16.1	16.7	17.3	17.9
Hiking, 40-lb pack, 3.0 MPH	4.1	4.5	4.9	5.3	5.7	6.1	6.5	6.9	7.3	7.7	8.1	8.5	8.9	9.3	9.7	10.1	10.5	10.9	11.3	11.7	12.1	12.5
Horseback riding (walk)	2.0	2.3	2.4	2.6	2.8	3.0	3.1	3.3	3.5	3.7	3.9	4.1	4.3	4.5	4.7	4.9	5.1	5.3	5.5	5.7	5.8	6.0
Horseback riding (trot)	4.1	4.4	4.8	5.2	5.6	6.0	6.4	6.8	7.2	7.6	8.0	8.4	8.8	9.2	9.6	10.0	10.4	10.8	11.2	11.6	12.0	12.4
Horseshoe pitching	2.1	2.3	2.5	2.7	3.0	3.3	3.4	3.6	3.8	4.0	4.2	4.4	4.6	4.8	5.0	5.2	5.4	5.6	5.8	6.0	6.3	6.5
Judo, karate	7.7	8.5	9.2	10.0	10.7	11.5	12.2	13.0	13.7	14.5	15.2	16.0	16.7	17.5	18.2	19.0	19.7	20.5	21.2	22.0	22.7	23.5
Mountain climbing	6.0	6.5	7.2	7.8	8.4	9.0	9.6	10.1	10.7	11.3	11.9	12.5	13.1	13.7	14.3	14.8	15.4	16.0	16.6	17.2	17.8	18.4
Paddleball, racquetball	5.9	6.4	7.0	7.6	8.1	8.7	9.3	9.9	10.4	11.0	11.6	12.1	12.7	13.3	13.9	14.4	15.0	15.6	16.1	16.7	17.3	17.9
Pool, billiards	1.1	1.2	1.3	1.4	1.5	1.6	1.7	1.8	1.9	2.0	2.1	2.2	2.4	2.5	2.6	2.7	2.8	2.9	3.0	3.1	3.2	3.3
Rope jumping 110 rpm	5.8	6.4	7.0	7.6	8.1	8.6	9.2	9.8	10.4	11.0	11.5	12.1	12.6	13.2	13.7	14.3	14.9	15.5	16.1	16.6	17.2	17.7
Rope jumping 120 rpm	5.6	6.1	6.7	7.2	7.7	8.3	8.8	9.4	9.9	10.5	11.0	11.5	12.1	12.6	13.1	13.7	14.3	14.8	15.4	15.9	16.4	17.0
Rope jumping 130 rpm	5.2	5.7	6.2	6.6	7.2	7.7	8.3	8.8	9.3	9.8	10.3	10.8	11.3	11.8	12.3	12.8	13.3	13.8	14.4	14.8	15.3	15.9
Rowing (recreation)	3.0	3.3	3.6	3.9	4.2	4.5	4.8	5.1	5.4	5.6	6.0	6.2	6.5	6.8	7.1	7.5	7.7	8.0	8.3	8.6	8.9	9.2
Rowing (machine)	8.2	9.0	9.8	10.6	11.4	12.2	13.0	13.8	14.6	15.4	16.2	17.0	17.8	18.6	19.4	20.2	21.0	21.8	22.6	23.4	24.2	25.0
Running, 11-min mile, 5.5 MPH	6.4	7.1	7.7	8.3	9.0	9.6	10.2	10.8	11.5	12.1	12.7	13.4	14.0	14.6	15.2	15.9	16.5	17.1	17.8	18.4	19.0	19.6

Appendix D—*Continued*

Body weight	90	99	108	117	125	134	143	152	161	170	178	187	196	205	213	222	231	240	249	257	266	275
Running, 8.5-min mile, 7 MPH	8.4	9.2	10.0	10.8	11.7	12.5	13.3	14.1	14.9	15.7	16.6	17.4	18.2	19.0	19.8	20.7	21.5	22.3	23.1	23.9	24.8	25.6
Running, 7-min mile, 9 MPH	9.3	10.2	11.1	12.9	13.1	13.9	14.8	15.7	16.6	17.5	18.9	19.3	20.2	21.1	22.1	23.0	23.9	24.8	25.7	26.6	27.5	28.4
Running, 5-min mile, 12 MPH	11.8	13.0	14.1	15.3	16.4	17.6	18.7	19.9	21.0	22.2	23.3	24.5	25.6	26.8	27.9	29.1	30.2	31.4	32.5	33.7	34.9	36.0
Stationary running, 140 counts/min	14.6	16.1	17.5	18.9	20.4	21.8	23.2	24.6	26.1	27.5	28.9	30.4	31.8	33.2	34.6	36.1	37.5	38.9	40.4	41.8	43.2	44.6
Sprinting	13.8	15.2	16.6	17.9	19.2	20.5	21.9	23.3	24.7	26.1	27.3	28.7	30.0	31.4	32.7	34.0	35.4	36.8	38.2	39.4	40.3	42.2
Sailing	1.8	2.0	2.1	2.3	2.4	2.7	2.8	3.0	3.2	3.4	3.6	3.8	3.9	4.1	4.3	4.4	4.6	4.8	5.0	5.1	5.3	5.5
Skating (moderate)	3.4	3.8	4.1	4.4	4.8	5.1	5.4	5.8	6.1	6.4	6.8	7.1	7.4	7.8	8.1	8.3	8.8	9.1	9.4	9.8	10.1	10.4
Skating (vigorous)	6.2	6.8	7.4	8.0	8.6	9.2	9.8	10.4	11.0	11.6	12.2	12.8	13.4	14.0	14.6	15.2	15.8	16.4	17.0	17.6	18.2	18.8
Skiing (downhill)	5.8	6.4	6.9	7.5	8.1	8.6	9.2	9.8	10.3	10.9	11.4	12.0	12.6	13.1	13.7	14.3	14.8	15.4	16.0	16.5	17.1	17.7
Skiing (level, 5 MPH)	7.0	7.7	8.4	9.1	9.8	10.5	11.1	11.8	12.5	13.2	13.9	14.6	15.2	15.9	16.6	17.3	18.0	18.7	19.4	20.0	20.7	21.4
Skiing (racing downhill)	9.9	10.9	11.9	12.9	13.7	14.7	15.7	16.7	17.7	18.7	19.6	20.6	21.6	22.6	23.4	24.4	25.4	26.4	27.4	28.3	29.3	30.2
Snowshoeing (2.3 MPH)	3.7	4.1	4.5	4.8	5.2	5.5	5.9	6.3	6.7	7.0	7.4	7.8	8.1	8.5	8.8	9.2	9.6	9.9	10.3	10.6	11.0	11.4
Snowshoeing (2.5 MPH)	5.4	5.9	6.5	7.0	7.5	8.0	8.6	9.1	9.7	10.2	10.7	11.2	11.8	12.3	12.8	13.3	13.9	14.4	14.9	15.4	16.0	16.5
Soccer	5.4	5.9	6.4	6.9	7.5	8.0	8.5	9.0	9.6	10.1	10.6	11.1	11.6	12.2	12.7	13.2	13.4	14.3	14.8	15.3	15.8	16.9
Squash	6.2	6.8	7.5	8.1	8.7	9.3	9.9	10.5	11.1	11.7	12.3	12.9	13.5	14.2	14.8	15.4	16.0	16.6	17.2	17.8	18.4	19.0
Stair climbing and descending:																						
1 stair—25 trips/min	4.1	4.5	4.9	5.3	5.6	6.0	6.4	6.8	7.2	7.7	8.0	8.4	8.8	9.2	9.6	10.0	10.4	10.8	11.2	11.6	12.0	12.4
1 stair—30 trips/min	4.4	4.9	5.3	5.7	6.1	6.6	7.0	7.4	7.9	8.3	8.7	9.2	9.6	10.0	10.4	10.9	11.3	11.8	12.2	12.6	13.0	13.5
1 stair—35 trips/min	5.0	5.5	6.0	6.6	7.0	7.5	8.0	8.5	9.0	9.5	10.0	10.5	11.0	11.5	11.9	12.4	12.9	13.4	13.9	14.4	14.9	15.4
3 stairs—12 trips/min	4.8	5.2	5.7	6.2	6.6	7.1	7.6	8.1	8.5	9.0	9.4	9.9	10.4	10.9	11.3	11.8	12.2	12.7	13.2	13.6	14.1	14.6

Appendix D—*Continued*

Body weight	90	99	108	117	125	134	143	152	161	170	178	187	196	205	213	222	231	240	249	257	266	275
3 stairs—15 trips/min	5.8	6.3	6.9	7.5	8.0	8.6	9.2	9.8	10.3	10.9	11.4	12.0	12.5	13.1	13.6	14.2	14.8	15.4	15.9	16.4	17.0	17.6
3 stairs—18 trips/min	6.8	7.4	8.1	8.8	9.4	10.1	10.7	11.4	12.1	12.8	13.4	14.0	14.7	15.4	16.0	16.7	17.3	18.0	18.7	19.3	20.0	20.6
5 stairs—8 trips/min	4.9	5.3	5.8	6.3	6.8	7.2	7.7	8.2	8.7	9.2	9.6	10.1	10.6	11.1	11.5	12.0	12.5	13.0	13.4	13.9	14.4	14.9
5 stairs—10 trips/min	6.0	6.6	7.2	7.8	8.4	9.0	9.6	10.2	10.8	11.4	11.9	12.5	13.1	13.7	14.3	14.9	15.5	16.1	16.7	17.2	17.8	18.4
5 stairs—12 trips/min	6.8	7.5	8.2	8.9	9.5	10.2	10.9	11.6	12.2	12.9	13.5	14.2	14.9	15.6	16.2	16.9	17.6	18.2	18.9	19.5	20.2	20.9
7 stairs—6 trips/min	5.1	5.6	6.2	6.7	7.1	7.7	8.2	8.7	9.2	9.7	10.1	10.7	11.2	11.7	12.1	12.7	13.2	13.7	14.2	14.6	15.2	15.7
7 stairs—7½ trips/min	6.1	6.7	7.3	8.0	8.5	9.1	9.7	10.3	10.9	11.6	12.1	12.7	13.3	13.9	14.5	15.1	15.7	16.3	16.9	17.5	18.1	18.7
7 stairs—9 trips/min	7.2	7.9	8.6	9.4	10.0	10.7	11.4	12.2	12.9	13.6	14.2	15.0	15.7	16.4	17.0	17.8	18.5	19.2	19.9	20.6	21.3	22.0
Swimming, pleasure 25 yds/min	3.6	4.0	4.3	4.7	5.0	5.4	5.7	6.1	6.4	6.8	7.1	7.5	7.8	8.2	8.5	8.9	9.2	9.6	10.0	10.3	10.6	11.0
Swimming, back 20 yds/min	2.3	2.6	2.8	3.0	3.2	3.5	3.7	3.9	4.1	4.2	4.6	4.8	5.0	5.3	5.5	5.7	6.0	6.2	6.4	6.6	6.9	7.1
Swimming, back 30 yds/min	3.2	3.5	3.8	4.1	4.4	4.7	5.1	5.4	5.7	6.0	6.3	6.6	6.9	7.2	7.4	7.9	8.2	8.5	8.8	9.1	9.4	9.7
Swimming, back 40 yds/min	5.0	5.5	5.8	6.5	7.0	7.5	7.9	8.5	8.9	9.4	9.9	10.4	10.9	11.4	11.9	12.3	12.8	13.3	13.8	14.3	14.8	15.3
Swimming, breast 20 yds/min	2.9	3.2	3.4	3.8	4.0	4.3	4.6	4.9	5.1	5.4	5.7	6.0	6.3	6.5	6.8	7.1	7.4	7.7	7.9	8.2	8.5	8.8
Swimming, breast 30 yds/min	4.3	4.8	5.2	5.7	6.0	6.4	6.9	7.3	7.7	8.1	8.6	9.0	9.4	9.9	10.3	10.8	11.1	11.5	11.9	12.4	13.0	13.3
Swimming, breast 40 yds/min	5.8	6.3	6.9	7.5	8.0	8.6	9.2	9.7	10.3	10.8	11.4	12.0	12.5	13.1	13.7	14.2	14.8	15.4	15.9	16.5	17.0	17.6
Swimming, butterfly 50 yds/min	7.0	7.7	8.4	9.1	9.8	10.5	11.1	11.9	12.5	13.2	13.9	14.6	15.2	15.9	16.6	17.3	18.0	18.7	19.4	20.0	20.7	21.4
Swimming, crawl 20 yds/min	2.9	3.2	3.4	3.8	4.0	4.3	4.6	4.9	5.1	5.4	5.7	5.8	6.3	6.5	6.8	7.1	7.3	7.7	7.9	8.2	8.5	8.8

Appendix D—*Continued*

Body weight	90	99	108	117	125	134	143	152	161	170	178	187	196	205	213	222	231	240	249	257	266	275
Swimming, crawl 45 yds/min	5.2	5.8	6.3	6.8	7.3	7.8	8.3	8.8	9.3	9.8	10.4	10.9	11.4	11.9	12.4	12.9	13.4	13.9	14.4	15.0	15.5	16.0
Swimming, crawl 50 yds/min	6.4	7.0	7.6	8.3	8.9	9.5	10.1	10.7	11.4	12.0	12.6	13.2	13.9	14.5	15.1	15.7	16.3	17.0	17.4	17.9	18.8	19.5
Table tennis	2.3	2.6	2.8	3.0	3.2	3.5	3.7	3.9	4.1	4.2	4.6	4.8	5.0	5.3	5.5	5.7	6.0	6.2	6.4	6.6	6.9	7.1
Tennis (recreation)	4.2	4.6	5.0	5.4	5.8	6.2	6.6	7.0	7.4	7.8	8.2	8.6	9.0	9.4	9.8	10.2	10.6	11.0	11.5	11.9	12.3	12.6
Tennis (competition)	5.9	6.4	7.0	7.6	8.1	8.7	9.3	9.9	10.4	11.0	11.6	12.1	12.7	13.3	13.9	14.4	15.0	15.6	16.1	16.7	17.3	17.9
Timed calisthenics	8.8	9.6	10.5	11.4	12.2	13.1	13.9	14.8	15.6	16.5	17.4	18.2	19.1	19.9	20.8	21.5	22.5	23.9	24.2	25.1	25.9	26.8
Vollyball (moderate)	3.4	3.8	4.0	4.4	4.8	5.1	5.4	5.8	6.1	6.4	6.8	7.1	7.4	7.8	8.1	8.3	8.8	9.1	9.4	9.8	10.1	10.4
Volleyball (vigorous)	5.9	6.4	7.0	7.6	8.1	8.7	9.3	9.9	10.4	11.0	11.6	12.1	12.7	13.3	13.9	14.4	15.0	15.6	16.1	16.7	17.3	17.9
Walking (2.0 MPH)	2.1	2.3	2.5	2.7	2.9	3.1	3.3	3.5	3.7	4.0	4.2	4.4	4.6	4.8	5.0	5.2	5.4	5.6	5.8	6.0	6.2	6.4
Walking (4.5 MPH)	4.0	4.4	4.7	5.1	5.5	5.9	6.3	6.7	7.1	7.5	7.8	8.2	8.6	9.0	9.4	9.8	10.1	10.6	10.9	11.3	11.7	12.0
Walking 110–120 steps/min	3.1	3.4	3.7	4.0	4.3	4.7	5.0	5.3	5.6	5.9	6.2	6.5	6.8	7.1	7.4	7.7	8.0	8.3	8.6	8.9	9.2	9.5
Waterskiing	4.7	5.1	5.6	6.1	6.5	7.0	7.4	7.9	8.3	8.8	9.3	9.7	10.2	10.6	11.1	11.5	12.0	12.5	12.9	13.4	13.8	14.3
Weight training	4.7	5.1	5.7	6.2	6.7	7.0	7.5	7.9	8.4	8.9	9.4	9.9	10.3	10.8	11.1	11.7	12.2	12.6	13.1	13.5	14.0	14.4
Wrestling	7.7	8.5	9.2	10.0	10.7	11.5	12.2	13.0	13.7	14.5	15.2	16.0	16.7	17.5	18.2	19.0	19.7	20.5	21.2	22.0	22.7	23.5
XBX, 5BX, Chart 1*	5.0	5.5	5.9	6.4	6.9	7.4	7.9	8.4	8.6	9.3	9.8	10.3	10.8	11.3	11.8	12.3	12.8	13.2	13.7	14.2	14.7	15.2
XBX, 5BX, Chart 2*	6.2	6.9	7.5	8.1	8.7	9.3	9.9	10.5	11.1	11.7	12.3	12.9	13.6	14.2	14.8	15.4	16.0	16.7	17.2	17.8	18.4	19.0
XBX, 5BX, Charts 3, 4*	8.8	9.6	10.5	11.4	12.2	13.1	13.9	14.8	15.6	16.5	17.4	18.2	19.1	19.9	20.8	21.6	22.5	23.4	24.2	25.1	25.9	26.8
5BX, Charts 5, 6*	10.0	10.9	11.9	12.9	13.9	14.9	15.8	16.8	17.8	18.7	19.7	20.7	21.7	22.6	23.6	24.6	25.5	26.7	27.4	28.1	29.4	30.1

*Canadian Ten Basic Exercise and Five Basic Exercise Programs in Royal Canadian Air Force, Royal Canadian Air Force Exercise Plans for Physical Fitness (New York: Essandess Special Editions), pp. 18, 24, 30, 36, 69, 71, 73, 75, 77, 79.

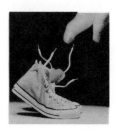

Suggested Readings

Age

Shepard, R. *Physical Activity and Aging.* Chicago: Year Book Medical Publishers, 1978.

Smith, E., and R. Serfass. *Exercise and Aging.* Hillside, N.J.: Enslow, 1981.

Tamaris, P. S. *Developmental Physiology and Aging.* New York: Macmillan, 1972.

Athletic Injuries

Anderson, J. L. *The Yearbook of Sports Medicine.* Chicago: Year Book Medical Publishers, 1981.

Mirkin, Gabe, and Marshall Hoffman. *Sports Medicine Book.* Boston: Little, Brown, 1978.

Olsen, O. C. *Prevention of Injuries, Protecting the Health of Student Athletes.* Philadelphia: Lea & Febiger, 1971.

Bicycling

Delong, Fred. *Delong's Guide to Bicycles and Bicycling.* Radnor, Penn.: Chilton, 1974.

Kingbay, Keith. *Inside Bicycling.* Chicago: Contemporary Books, 1977.

Sloane, Eugene A. *The New Complete Book of Bicycling.* New York: Simon & Schuster, 1974.

Cross-Country Skiing

Caldwell, John. *New Cross-Country Ski Book.* 4th ed. Brattleboro, Vt.: Greene, 1973.

Gillette, Ned. *Cross-Country Skiing with John Dostal.* Seattle: The Mountaineers, 1979.

Thronton, Pat. *Contemporary Cross-Country Skiing.* Chicago: Chicago Books, 1978.

Heart Disease

American Heart Association Handbook. New York: E. P. Dulton, 1980.

Fisher, Arthur. *The Healthy Heart.* Chicago: Time-Life Books, 1981.

Friedman, Meyer, and Ray H. Rosenman. *Type A Behavior and Your Heart.* Greenwich, Conn.: Fawcett, 1974.

Halhuber, Canula, and Max Halhuber. *Speaking of Heart Attacks.* New York: Consolidated Book Publisher, 1978.

Pollock, Michael, and Donald Schmidt. *Heart Disease and Rehabilitation.* Boston: Houghton Mifflin, 1979.

Solomon, Henry A. *The Exercise Myth.* New York: Harcourt Brace Jovanovich, 1984.

Zohman, Lenore. *The Cardiologist's Guide to Fitness and Health through Excellence.* New York: Simon & Schuster, 1979.

Nutrition and Weight Control

Briggs, George M., and Doris H. Calloway. *Bogert's Nutrition and Physical Fitness.* Philadelphia: Saunders, 1979.

Brody, Jane. *Jane Brody's Nutrition Book.* New York: Norton, 1981.

Guthrie, Helen. *Introductory Nutrition.* St. Louis: C. V. Mosby, 1983.

Katch, Frank I., and William D. McArdle. *Nutrition, Weight Control and Exercise.* Boston: Houghton Mifflin, 1977.

Whitney, Eleanor N., and Corinne B. Cataldo. *Understanding Normal and Clinical Nutrition.* St. Paul: West, 1983.

Orienteering

Disley, John. *Orienteering.* Harrisburg, Penn.: Stackpole Books, 1969.

Kjellstrom, Bjorn. *Be Expert with Map and Compass, The Orienteering Handbook.* New York: Charles Scribner & Sons, 1976.

Physical Fitness and Health

Allsen, Phillip E., Joyce M. Harrison, and Barbara Vance. *Fitness for Life.* 3d ed. Dubuque, Iowa: Wm. C. Brown, 1984.

Cooper, Kenneth. *Aerobics.* New York: Evans, 1969.

Corbin, Charles and Ruth Lindsy. *Concepts of Physical Fitness with Laboratory.* 5th ed. Dubuque, Iowa: Wm. C. Brown, 1985.

Di Gennaro, Joseph. *The New Physical Fitness: Exercise for Every Body.* Englewood, Colo.: Morton, 1983.

Dintiman, George B., Stephan E. Stone, Jude C. Pennington, and Robert G. Davis. *Discovering Lifetime Fitness.* St. Paul: West, 1984.

Falls, Arnold B., Ann M. Baylor, and Rud K. Dishman. *Essentials of Fitness.* Philadelphia: Saunders, 1980.

Getchell, Bud. *Physical Fitness, A Way of Life.* 3d ed. New York: Wiley, 1983.

Marley, William. *Health and Physical Fitness.* Philadelphia: Saunders, 1982.

Pollock, Michael, Jack H. Wilmore, and Samuel M. Fox. *Exercise in Health and Disease.* Philadelphia: Saunders, 1984.

Rosensweig, S. *Sports Fitness for Women.* New York: Harper & Row, 1982.

Physiology of Exercise

Brooks, George A., and Thomas D. Fahey. *Exercise Physiology.* New York: John Wiley & Sons, 1984.

Devries, Herbert A. *Physiology of Exercise for Physical Education and Athletics.* 3d ed. Philadelphia: Saunders, 1980.

Fox, E. L. *Sports Physiology.* Philadelphia: Saunders, 1979.

Lamb, David R. *Physiology of Exercise.* New York: Macmillan, 1984.

Shaver, Larry G. *Essentials of Exercise Physiology.* Minneapolis: Burgess, 1981.

Wilmore, Jack H. *Training for Sport and Activity, The Physiological Basis of Conditioning.* 2d ed. Boston: Allyn & Bacon, 1982.

Running

Anderson, Bob. *Stretching*. Bolinas, Calif.: Shelton, 1980.

Costill, David L. *A Scientific Approach to Distance Running*. Los Altos, Calif.: Track and Field News, 1979.

Daniels, Jack, Robert Fitts, and George Sheehan. *Conditioning for Distance Runners*. New York: Wiley, 1978.

Fix, James F. *The Complete Book of Running*. New York: Random House, 1977.

Fix, James F. *Second Book of Running*. New York: Random House, 1980.

Galloway, Jeff. *Galloway's Book on Running*. Bolinas, Calif.: Shelton, 1984.

Glasser, William. *Positive Addiction*. New York: Harper & Row, 1976.

Sheehan, George. *Running and Being*. New York: Simon & Schuster, 1978.

Smith, Nathan J. *Food for Sport*. Palo Alto, Calif.: Bull, 1976.

Ullyot, Joan. *Running Free*. New York: G. P. Putman & Sons, 1982.

Sports Activities

Kisselle, D., and K. Mazzou. *Aerobic Dance: A Way to Fitness*. Denver, Colo.: Morton, 1983.

Penrod, James, and Janice Plastine. *The Dancer Prepares: Modern Dance for Beginners*. Palo Alto, Calif.: Mayfield, 1970.

Sorensen, Jackie. *Aerobic Dancing*. New York: Rawson Wade, 1979.

Vincent, L. M. *The Dancer's Book of Health*. Kansas City, Kan.: Sheed Andrews & McMeel, 1978.

Strength and Muscle Development

Darden, Ellington. *The Nautilus Book*. Chicago: Contemporary Books, 1982.

Darden, Ellington. *The Nautilus Woman*. New York: Simon & Schuster, 1983.

Fox, E. L., and D. K. Mathews. *Interval Training, Conditioning for Sport and General Fitness*. Philadelphia: Saunders, 1974.

Jarrell, Steve. *Working Out with Weights*. New York: Anco, 1982.

Kirkley, George W. *Weight Lifting and Weight Training*. New York: Anco, 1981.

Leon, Edie. *Complete Woman Weight Training Guide*. Mountain View, Calif.: Anderson World, 1976.

O'Shea, J. P. *Scientific Principles and Methods of Strength Fitness*. Reading, Mass.: Addison-Wesley, 1979.

Sobey, Edwin. *Strength Training Book*. Mountain View, Calif.: Anderson World, 1981.

Westcott, Wayne. *Strength Fitness, Physiological Principles and Training Techniques*. Boston: Allyn & Bacon, 1982.

Swimming

Counsilman, James E. *The Complete Book of Swimming*. New York: Atheneum, 1977.

Midtlyng, Joanna. *Swimming*. Philadelphia: Saunders, 1974.

Testing and Evaluation

Golding, Lawrence A., Clayton R. Meyers, and Wayne E. Sinning. *The Y's Way to Physical Fitness*. Rosemont, Ill.: National Board of YMCA, 1982.

Pollock, Michael, Jack Wilmore, and Samuel M. Fox. *Health and Fitness through Physical Activity*. Philadelphia: Saunders, 1984.

Wilson, Phil, ed. *Adult Fitness and Cardiac Rehabilitation*. Baltimore: University Park Press, 1975.

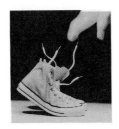

Index